SPORTS OFFICIALS AND OFFICIATING

T0262598

Sports officials (umpires, referees, judges) play a vital role in every sport, and sports governing bodies, fans, and players now expect officials to maintain higher professional standards than ever before. In this ground-breaking book, a team of leading international sport scientists and top level officials have come together to examine, for the first time, the science and practice of officiating in sport, helping us to better understand the skills, techniques, and physical requirements of successful refereeing.

The book covers every key component of the official's role, including:

- Training and career development
- Fitness and physical preparation
- Visual processing
- Judgement and decision making
- Communication and game management
- Psychological demands and skills
- Using technology
- Performance evaluation
- Researching and studying officials in sport

Top-level officials or officiating managers contribute in the 'Official's Call' sections, reflecting on their experiences in real in-game situations across a wide range of international sports, and on how a better understanding of science and technique can help improve professional practice. No other book has attempted to combine leading edge contemporary sport science with the realities of match officiating in this way, and therefore this book is vital reading for any advanced student of sport science, sport coaching or sport development, or any practising official or sports administrator looking to raise their professional standards.

Clare MacMahon Head of Sports Science at Swinburne University of Technology in Melbourne, Australia

Duncan Mascarenhas British Psychological Society Chartered Psychologist, Senior Lecturer at Glyndŵr University, Wrexham, UK

Henning Plessner PhD in Psychology, Professor for Sport Psychology and Director of the Institute of Sports and Sports Sciences at the University of Heidelberg, Germany

Alexandra Pizzera Post-Doctoral Fellow at the Institute of Psychology of the German Sport University Cologne

Raôul R. D. Oudejans Associate Professor at the MOVE Research Institute Amsterdam, Faculty of Human Movement Sciences, VU University, The Netherlands

Markus Raab Head of the Institute of Psychology at the German Sport University and Head of the Performance Psychology Department, and Research Professor at London South Bank University, UK

SPORTS OFFICIALS AND OFFICIATING

Science and practice

Clare MacMahon, Duncan Mascarenhas, Henning Plessner, Alexandra Pizzera, Raôul R. D. Oudejans and Markus Raab

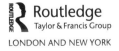

LONDON AND NEW YORK

First published 2015
by Routledge
2 Park Square, Milton Park, Abingdon, Oxon OX14 4RN

and by Routledge
711 Third Avenue, New York, NY 10017

Routledge is an imprint of the Taylor & Francis Group, an informa business

© 2015 Clare MacMahon, Duncan Mascarenhas, Henning Plessner,
Alexandra Pizzera, Raôul R. D. Oudejans and Markus Raab

British Library Cataloguing-in-Publication Data
A catalogue record for this book is available from the British Library

Library of Congress Cataloging-in-Publication Data
MacMahon, Clare.
Sports officials and officiating : science and practice/Clare MacMahon,
Duncan Mascarenhas, Henning Plessner, Alexandra Pizzera,
Ra?ul R.D. Oudejans and Markus Raab.
pages cm
Includes bibliographical references and index.
1. Sports officiating—Handbooks, manuals, etc. 2. Sports officials—
Training of. I. Title.
GV735.M33 2015
796.023—dc23
2014021704

ISBN: 978-0-415-83574-9 (hbk)
ISBN: 978-0-415-83575-6 (pbk)
ISBN: 978-0-203-70052-5 (ebk)

Typeset in Bembo
by Swales & Willis Ltd, Exeter, Devon, UK

Printed and bound in the United States of America by Publishers Graphics,
LLC on sustainably sourced paper.

CONTENTS

CONTRIBUTORS

Clare MacMahon is Head of Sports Science at Swinburne University of Technology in Melbourne, Australia. Her research broadly examines movement cognition, exploring how thinking and moving are interlinked, with examples such as the impact of cognitive fatigue on physical performance or the impact of context on decisions in sport. Clare has also worked with a number of professional sporting organisations understanding talent identification and development, and training of cognitive skills such as decision making. She has worked with officials in a multitude of sports, at a variety of different levels in both research and application.

Duncan Mascarenhas is a British Psychological Society Chartered Psychologist with over 15 years of experience working with sports officials. Having provided psychological support to the Rugby Football Union Elite Referee Unit, he has since provided training to many clients including the Rugby Football League Match Officials and New Zealand Netball. He completed a post-doctoral research project with New Zealand Soccer referees investigating the interactive effect of physical performance and decision making. Duncan is a UK level 4 basketball referee and currently enjoys refereeing basketball, touch-rugby and soccer. He is currently employed at Glyndŵr University as a Senior Lecturer in Sport and Exercise Psychology. Duncan is a BASES (British Association of Sport & Exercise Sciences) Accredited Sport & Exercise Scientist and has research interests in team decision making, sports officiating and video interventions in sport.

Henning Plessner, PhD in Psychology, is Professor for Sport Psychology and Director of the Institute of Sports and Sports Sciences at the University of Heidelberg, Germany. The focus of his theoretical and empirical research work is on the experimental investigation of basic processes of social judgement, as well as on the study of judgement and decision making in various applied settings.

Henning is Vice-President of the German Society of Sport Science and the author/editor of three books, three journal special issues and more than 50 peer-reviewed articles and edited book chapters. Besides, he has been active as a national certified gymnastic judge for more than 20 years.

Alexandra Pizzera is a Post-Doctoral Fellow at the Institute of Psychology of the German Sport University Cologne where she also completed her Diploma degree in Sport Science and her PhD in Sport Science (Sport Psychology). Her research interests focus on the bidirectional link between action and perception with regard to visual and acoustic perception, expertise research and the selection, training and performance evaluation process of sports officials. She teaches courses in sport psychology and gymnastics.

Raôul R. D. Oudejans is Associate Professor at the MOVE Research Institute Amsterdam, Faculty of Human Movement Sciences, VU University, The Netherlands. His main research and teaching areas are perceiving and moving in sports (including sports officiating) and other high-pressure contexts, with emphasis on the psychological factors involved in performing. For the last 15 years Raôul has specialised in the visual control of the basketball shot as well as in training and performing under pressure. He has published over 60 peer-reviewed papers, eight book chapters and four books, including the new student book in Dutch *Sportpsychologie (Sport Psychology)* first published in 2012.

Markus Raab is the Head of the Institute of Psychology at the German Sport University and the Head of the Performance Psychology Department. Additionally, he is Research Professor at London South Bank University, UK. The main focus of the research programme in performance psychology is on motor learning and motor control and judgement and decision making in sports and beyond. He favours a simple heuristic approach and an embodied cognition approach to understanding the interaction of sensorimotor and cognitive behaviour from a psychological perspective.

Officials

Holger Albrecht, Federation International de Gymnastique (FIG) Technical Committee Member for Men's Artistic Gymnastics, Germany

Wayne Barnes, International Rugby Board (IRB) Referee, England

Ralf Brand, Referee and Member of Referee's Advisory Board, Basketball Bundesliga (BEKO BBL), Germany

Janie Frampton, Former National Referee Manager, the Football Association (FA), England

Graham Hughes, International Rugby Board (IRB) Television Match Official (TMO), England

Marika Humphreys-Baranova, International Skating Union (ISU) Judge, ISU Trainer and Examiner of Technical Specialists, England

Jacqui Jashari, International Netball Umpire; Umpire coach and mentor, Australia

Tom Lopes, Executive Director of International Association of Approved Basketball Officials (IAABO), USA

Bill Mildenhall, Referee Development Officer, Basketball Victoria and Victorian Basketball Referees Association, Australia

Tony Parker, International Squash Official, England

Chris White, Rugby Football Union (RFU) Referee Academy Manager, England

PREFACE

In July 2009, in a very hot Tucson, Arizona, the National Association of Sports Officials (NASO) held their annual summit. The topic was 'Judgment and Decision Making: How Officiating Leaders Make Great Calls'. A few months earlier I had found a review by NASO founder and *Referee* magazine publisher and executive editor Barry Mano on a book I co-edited on sport expertise,[1] with a chapter on the sports official.[2] I wrote to Barry to gain access to the article and, after a few correspondences back and forth, was on the NASO summit keynote speaker list. Among the speakers were extremely high-profile US officials who had refereed numerous Super Bowls, NCAA basketball finals, Stanley Cups – people who might easily find video clips of themselves on ESPN.

It was very important for NASO to have assurances that I would be an engaging speaker and not just a dry academic presenting graphs and statistics. I was asked to provide a reference to support my speaking skills. This isn't something academics are used to – we listen to boring talks all the time. We ask people to present research hoping they'll be engaging, but are sometimes unsurprised if they aren't. I was also the only academic at the summit presenting and talking about research with and about officiating. I was excited about the talk, and the opportunity to present research to an audience of officials interested in developing their skills and addressing critical topics. And decision making with officials is a topic right up my alley. I felt like a kid in a candy shop told to choose only a few candies from a massive and enticing selection. I wanted to present everything to them, with depth.

This experience, and those that each co-author of this book has whenever we speak to officiating groups, clearly showed us the need to write a book that bridges the science and the practice in sports officiating. We feel as though there is so much to tell – but it must be told in the right way. We are research geeks – excited by formulating and testing hypotheses, finding statistical significance, and reporting important advances to theory. But we are *applied researchers* who are driven by improving performance. We ask questions like: "Does it matter where the assistant referee stands to make decisions?", "What if we teach referees to fake penalties themselves in soccer to improve their ability to pick up deception?" and "Does seeing a really poor gymnastics performance make the next one look that much better?". So we like to think we're cool geeks, if that's possible, getting into the nitty gritty and exploring a cool topic that can have direct application. The areas we research are often as interesting to us as the casual sports fan next to us in the bar watching the game. More importantly, the research in which we are engaged can be influential for officials – for how they train, how they perform and how they are assessed.

It's clear to us that sports officials have always been in the shadow of athletes and coaches. This is often purposeful, and of great benefit to their role. One way it does not benefit them, however, is that they receive substantially less attention from sport science when it comes to understanding and improving performance. Rule books and technical guides help communicate the explicit knowledge that officials need. There has been little or no attempt, however, to communicate research that investigates the science behind accepted practice or suspected effects. This is our goal here. What we need is effective communication without losing the depth.

Specifically, the aim of this book is to bring together the growing research on sports officiating in a way that is empirically based, but also accessible to officials and administrators working 'at the coal face'. The chapters that follow review the science behind the development, training and performance of officials, covering specific research on areas like vision and decision making, communication, technology and psychological skills. We discuss interesting findings such as the influence of the colour an athlete competes in, why a decision early in a game is different from a decision later in a game and how an official's past history as an athlete can influence his/her development and performance.

The intention of this book is to address sports officiating as a collective. Although it is driven by the research, and thus may emphasise particular types of officials when this is the population the research has used (e.g. soccer referees), it is aimed at all sports, with application for the gymnastics judge as much as the football referee and the tennis line judge. It presents information that is of interest to the developing recreational official, the elite official, the officiating trainer and evaluator, as well as administrators designing programmes. This approach facilitates information sharing across sports and across sport roles, where lessons are learned, analogies are formed and advances are made.

We have organised the book emphasising our perspective of the importance of perceptual-cognitive skills of officials and including the topics that are most current in the sport science research in officiating. We have also included areas where there is less direct research with officials, like psychological skills and technology, but that are undoubtedly applicable. The chapters that follow emphasise research in the area but communicate this work in a way that is accessible to both researchers and practitioners. We have tried to limit weighty jargon, graphs and statistics, and have used a numbered referencing style to provide a path for readers who would like to delve further without bogging down those who are focused on gaining a more general understanding of the science behind sports officiating. To break things up, we have also used text boxes to include related but less central topics, interesting examples or illustrations of an effect or phenomenon or to illustrate tools or techniques referred to in the chapter.

Although all of us are or have been keen athletes and performers in a variety of sports including gymnastics, basketball, soccer, volleyball and rugby, we still wanted to ensure that the voice and view of the practitioner is included. To do this, each chapter concludes with a section called 'Official's Call'. These brief sections involve mostly high profile officials with experience relevant to the chapter topic. These officials were invited to provide critical reflection, experience and comment, as well as any specific examples of programming, practices and activities that relate to the topic. They did this in a variety of ways; many wrote the sections themselves after reading the chapters, or provided us with interviews from which we sourced their comments.

Our intention with this book is to provide a key resource for officials, officiating managers and trainers and sport administrators, given its practical emphasis. Yet we also aim to satisfy sport scientists, given our reliance on empirical evidence. We hope we have provided a 'first stop' reference for both the 'front line' officials and administrators and the 'back room' researchers delving into this area. In this way, we can bring researchers and officials together and avoid the view that research involves boring academics with no sense of the 'real world', or that officiating involves jocks with no interest in what they can gain from science.

Clare MacMahon, January 2014

[1] Farrow, D., Baker, J., & MacMahon, C. (Eds) (2008). *Developing sport expertise: Researchers and coaches put theory into practice.* London: Routledge.

[2] MacMahon, C., & Plessner, H. (2008). The sports official in research and practice. In D. Farrow, J. Baker, & C. MacMahon (Eds). *Developing sport expertise: Researchers and coaches put theory into practice* (pp. 172–92). London: Routledge.

ACKNOWLEDGEMENTS

We would like to thank a number of people who have helped contribute to this book. First, we acknowledge the numerous officials who were generous enough to provide comments and perspectives in their Official's Call sections. For help with materials, we also acknowledge Daniel Chalkley, Marika Vertzonis and Melanie Nash. Mark Sheeky generously contributed photographs, for which we are grateful. Finally, we thank Brendan Major for his editorial help with formatting for the chapters.

1

INTRODUCTION

A Google search for 'sport science and athlete' yields 50,200,000 results. In comparison, searching for 'sport science and referee' yields 26,200,000 results and 'sport science and officiating' yields only 243,000 results. This is not a rigorous comparison and does not account for how relevant each result is for the topics we'd like to compare, which is research on sports officials versus research on sports athletes. Nevertheless, it reflects what we know is true about these areas: there is far more research on athletes than there is on officials. In general this is not surprising when we consider the numbers: there are more athletes than there are officials. In other ways, however, the extent of the imbalance *is* surprising, given the impact that officials have on the outcome of contests.

One factor that creates a barrier to researching officials as a group is the diversity of the role; there are many different types of officials and a variety of specific demands. We only have to consider the soccer referee next to the gymnastics judge and the tennis linesperson to appreciate the variety of officials. This breadth is clear when we look at the Sport and Recreation New Zealand (SPARC) definition of an official as 'any person who controls the actual play of a competition by using the rules and laws of the sport to make judgments on rule infringement, performance, time and score. Officials play a key role in ensuring the spirit of the game and/or event is observed by all.'[1] There are a large number of different skills required to control a competition and ensure the spirit of the game, as described by SPARC: 'Sports officials must be able to bring control to chaos, understand fairness, promote safety, and encourage good sportsmanship. A sports official must have the positive characteristics of a police officer, lawyer, judge, accountant, reporter, athlete, and diplomat.'

Chapter 2 in this text addresses the diversity of officials specifically, introducing the three main types that are referred to throughout the book (interactors, monitors and reactors). This chapter also proposes an adapted model of the different developmental pathways and provides labels for officials at the different stages (e.g., the bread and butter official). The specific stage, category or type of official has an impact on factors such as motives, goals and training, which are all discussed in Chapter 2.

The broad-based understanding of officials as a group, provided in Chapter 2, serves as a foundation to presenting more specific areas of research with this population. Examining the research shows that, in general, the sports official holds a unique place in science. Perhaps due to the variety and complexity of different possible roles as well as the multiple factors at play in officiating, key research on officials that informs practice can be found in areas as diverse as psychology, economics, statistics and mathematics, management and sociology. While we argue that there is still limited research overall with officials, it is interesting to trace research themes over time to gain a sense of the evolution of focus with this population. In early work the emphasis appears to have been bias, personality factors and stress. The focus then transitioned to training activities, including physiological measurement, expert–novice differences and perceptual-cognitive abilities such as judgement and decision making. Areas such as game management and communication, vision and decision training became a focus, as well as management practices, injury, self-efficacy, gender and recruiting and retention trends. Again, these transitions over the last fifty or so years show an acknowledgement of the demands and tasks of the official, an appreciation of the specifics of particular roles and a more sophisticated understanding. Our goal in this book in the main chapters is to bring together and provide an overview of some of the most central findings.

What is also noticeable when perusing the published research on officials is the consistent presence of the topic of stress. The type of stress varies, however, as highlighted in a recent article which categorises five main sources:[2]

- competing responsibilities (e.g., family, training time) leading to time stress
- a lack of recognition on both an individual performance level and in the role of officials in general
- fear of physical harm from spectators and players
- performance stress and worry about making errors
- worry over conflict with other officials, competitors, and coaches.

This list coincides well with the key areas we review in the chapters that follow: training, development and motivation, perception, management and communication. Our perspective and, hence, emphasis in this book is from the parent disciplines of Psychology, Human Movement and Education. We therefore emphasise the cognitive aspects of officiating – from learning and decision making to factors that have an impact on recruiting, performance and retention. This is often also referred to as expertise research, an area most of us would identify as at least part of our research focus.

An examination of the current edition of the *Handbook of Sports Psychology*,[3] which is a close match to our discipline focus as researchers and which emphasises athletes, shows how multifaceted sports psychology is, in general. It also shows how limited is the research with officials, and how far behind that with athletes. This is evident because many of the topics in the handbook that are examined in athletes are not touched on with as great depth – if at all –with officials. Specifically, the handbook includes main sections, with multiple chapters in each section, on:

- motivation, emotion and psychophysiology
- social perspectives (with chapters on leadership and self-presentation)
- sport expertise, outlining skill acquisition, anticipation and attention
- interventions and performance enhancement, with eight chapters covering mental skills, sports injury, choking and pre-shot routines
- physical activity and health psychology covering areas such as burnout and mental health
- life span development, outlining topics such as career transitions and termination
- methodological and measurement issues in research.

An additional special topics section covers disability, alcohol and drug abuse, and gender and cultural diversity. Again, many of these topics are relevant to officials but have not been researched with this population. For this reason, at this stage of the research with sports officials, these areas are used as a general base of knowledge for officials. We have selected, however, to emphasise the most central concerns from the expertise and cognitive perspectives. Hence, our chapters cover eight core topics (Chapters 2–9).

The acknowledgement of differences between officials from Chapter 2 leads us into the research on physical demands and evaluation. Chapter 3 acknowledges that many officials have high physical demands, outlining the training and evaluation of officials. The pervasive use of Global Positioning Systems (GPS) to track activity patterns has led to a much more detailed knowledge about the on-field distances covered by officials (emphasising soccer referees as the most studied group) and the type of activity used (e.g., running, walking). This information has in turn helped to drive training programmes. Chapter 3 presents these data, discusses how fitness is measured, and presents information on the relationship between physical demands/fitness and decision making.

Chapter 4 focuses on an area we often think of as the heart of officiating – vision and visual perception. We review the fascinating research around vision and the sports official, and how this can have an impact on the decisions that are made. We discuss the process of deciding what to take in and pay attention to, as well as how positioning can lead to errors of perception and thus judgement. This leads in to a discussion of practical suggestions and training for this skill. Again, this chapter emphasises the soccer referee as the role most often examined in the research.

The extensive work on judgement and decision making in sports officials is presented next, in Chapter 5. Here we move beyond perception and attention and distracting cues, as discussed in Chapter 4, and concentrate on the steps of information processing from the knowledge that lies under decisions, to how the information in the environment is perceived, then categorised and integrated with this knowledge to result in a decision. We touch on the impact of colour and home ground on decisions.

A key area that has emerged in acknowledging the complexity of the official's role is that of game management. This is central to the interactor official and involves communication with players and coaching personnel (and parents and spectators). As one of what may be referred to as 'intangible' or soft skills that are critical and can make or break an official, game management and communication is worthy of the attention it receives in Chapter 6. While Chapter 5 discusses the biases that can arise from context, Chapter 6 acknowledges that the use of context is often an essential skill in decision making and communication. Officiating style and philosophy are discussed, as is the key communication construct of corporate theatre.

Psychological skills, as a search for journal articles on officiating reveals, are critical in officiating. Chapter 7 tackles this area and emphasises mental skills such as self-talk, imagery and pre-event routines. A highlight of this chapter is its applied nature, setting out, for example, guidance on appropriate features of successful goal-setting.

The last few decades have seen a dramatic increase in both the use and the potential use of technology in sports officiating. As Chapter 8 points out, however, technology use in sports officiating has been around since automated timing was introduced. Moreover, there is a danger that spectators believe technology is immune to error. To gain some perspective on how technology can be used, this chapter reviews methods which are used to complement and contribute to officials' decisions, and those which replace the official as judge and decision maker.

Chapter 9 takes the preceding chapters into account and presents the training implications. It also outlines issues in the recruitment, selection and evaluation of officials. It touches on coping with the stress that officials inevitably experience, increasing the volume of decision making encountered by using video-based training, and methods and models used in the difficult task of evaluating performance.

A final concluding chapter reviews the themes and overall messages from the preceding chapters, and provides perspective on the state of the field and the next evolution for needed advancements in research on sports officiating for practice. As a whole, we anticipate that some of the findings and conclusions presented in this book will be unsurprising to practitioners, prompting responses that indicate 'we've always known this'. We see this as a positive, showing the coherence of the research with practice. We also see, however, that officiating research is developing and is beginning to move to more informative stages, as we discuss in Chapter 10. The further development of the field is shown in the studies presented throughout the book that go beyond confirming what has previously been known, and move to more informative and sometimes surprising findings. In fact, it is the combination of useful theory as well as practice that defines a finding that has impact. The entire field will soon arrive at this stage. Chapter 10 provides some perspective on questions and research that have both theoretical or discipline impact, as well as applied impact.

As a concluding point in introducing this text, we acknowledge the barriers to research in officiating from both the practitioner's (officiating manager and/or officials themselves) and the researcher's perspective. These are the barriers that contribute to the smaller volume of work compared to that with athletes, and are outlined in Table 1.1

As the table indicates, the researcher's primary goal in conducting officiating research is generally a greater understanding of a particular phenomenon or of human functioning. For example, the researcher might want to gain a better understanding of how context influences judgement in a complex task. The sports official provides an excellent task and population for this question. While research may then contribute to performance, in many cases this contribution is a side benefit from the researcher's point of view. This is not to say that researchers are not concerned with improving performance, and for many this can even be one of the primary goals. Research must also contribute to the general knowledge base, however, and while academic models emphasise publication of papers that have an impact on both theory and practice, many publication outlets emphasise theory and statistical significance much more so.

In contrast to the researcher, a practitioner's primary interest in research is to improve performance and maximise training. This may sometimes take the shape of statistical analyses which confirm current practices or management. With such a broad goal, practitioners may have difficulty identifying the right question, knowing what to ask (you don't know what you don't know), or at least prioritising one area for improvement. The time pressure for insights, improvements or the knowledge that will contribute to improvements is also high; practitioners are often primarily interested in quick feedback and short term outcomes. For example, taking on a new training programme is expected to show outcomes in the current season to support its ongoing use into the next season, particularly if it is novel and/or necessitates resources or 'buy in'.

A practitioner may want a researcher to express certainty in a programme and its impact or results, and to implement programmes across the board in the simplest

TABLE 1.1 The main barriers to officiating research

Stakeholder	Primary goals	Time pressures	Outcome timelines	Barriers
Researcher	Greater understanding	Low	Medium to long term	Funding, access to participants, 'good' questions
Practitioner	Improved performance	High	Short term	Funding, time, people, 'good' questions

manner possible, which requires fewer resources and less disruption. A researcher, on the other hand, may wish to be cautious in interpreting results and consider the scientific method such as sample size and generalisability. Researchers are also concerned with rigorous testing to contribute to greater certainty in their results, and with methods such as the use of treatment and control groups or multiple measures, which increase their chances of being published. These design features, however, may decrease the ease of implementation for practitioners and how viable it is to do the work at all.

Researchers have high time pressures on a day-to-day basis and are often balancing/juggling supervision, teaching, research and administration, but research activities are often 'slow burning' projects with regard to outcomes for results and publication. In contrast to the practitioner, the researcher is accustomed to incremental gains in knowledge and progress: many research projects are completed over a number of years with progressive steps and may involve multiple information sources such as experiments, database analyses and questionnaires. Publications often take up to several years from first submission to print. Researcher outcome timelines for research are thus medium to long term.

Although there are contrasting goals, interests and timelines, the barriers to participation in research on officiating for the researcher and the practitioner are similar, and often come down to resources and role-based priorities. Researchers often need to prioritise funded research within the university model and, if there is no funding or access to participants, the priority of a project with officials drops. Instead, researchers may find more funding or access to athletes or other populations with complex tasks that can serve to help in understanding phenomena or complex human functioning (e.g., emergency services).

Lack of funding for officiating research often stems from the priority placed by National Sporting Organisations on other activities. It may be that officiating itself is underfunded for a sport, and any research would have to be supported from an already meagre allowance. Or it may be that there is a specific research budget for a sport but work with athletes is prioritised. The lack of funding for research with officials from 'the sport side' is mirrored in 'the science side': funding bodies such as national level health and medical research councils or social or generalised government research councils often prioritise theory or application to areas such as medicine and general health principles. In many ways these funding bodies dictate the research topic, which either involves movement away from applied sport and officials or creative packaging of a topic where officiating is an analogy (e.g., sports participation for health). This means that 'good questions' that are of theoretical, fundable and also applied interest can be a barrier to working with officials.

For practitioners, funding resources are also a problem. However, a greater resource issue is human resources in the form of a sport liaison or expert collaborator (e.g., providing correct options on video tasks, encouraging participation, reviewing study designs, navigating the sporting organisation), or in access to officials as study participants. Because the outcomes of the research may not be immediate, the priority to dedicate these resources – and particularly to commit to complex research designs – may drop.

We propose that the identified barriers and their impact on the ability to ask 'good questions' from both a scientific and practical perspective have inhibited the growth of research on officials. As a result, there is an abundance of 'one-off' scattered studies on officiating. There are only a handful of structured ongoing programmes and few researchers with series of studies. Because we humbly suggest that we are among the researchers who have contributed more substantially to the area, it is our hope that the chapters that follow can be used to stimulate both the researcher and practitioner in formulating and asking interesting questions. We hope this helps to agitate for and create creative ways to access resources (people, time and funding) for research. We see this text as a tool for communication and dissemination, and a stimulus for continued thought and development. Ultimately, we hope this continued thought and development will generate interesting work that has an impact on important questions that influence both theory and practice. This is the challenge we put to you as you read on.

References

[1] Sport and Recreation New Zealand (SPARC). (2012). *Officials*. New Zealand: Sport and Recreation New Zealand. http://www.sparc.org.nz/en-nz/Information-For/ Officials/ (accessed 7 January 2014).

[2] Cuskelly, G., & Hoye, R. (2013). Sports officials' intention to continue. *Sport Management Review*, 16, 451–64.

[3] Tenenbaum, G., & Ekland, R.C. (Eds). (2007). *Handbook of Sport Psychology 3rd Edition*. New Jersey: John Wiley & Sons, Inc.

2

DEVELOPMENT OF OFFICIALS

Introduction

There's a fantastic television commercial in which a National Football League (NFL) umpire is standing on the side lines looking forward at the game play with an expressionless face. This is remarkable when the camera zooms out and you see the irate coach standing next to him shouting in his ear, inches away and jumping up and down. The game announcer is heard over the top of the scene saying "He's beating him like a rented mule! And the ref is just taking it. Boy, where do you train to take a beating like that?" The scene next switches to one in which the referee is in the exact same posture, with the exact same neutral expression, but the coach has been replaced by his wife who is yelling at him just as heatedly: " . . . when is that porch going to be painted? And that letter box? It's been three weeks? Three weeks!", she screeches.

The commercial raises a good question, and perhaps presents even better ones about where and how people train to become officials, and why someone would take on a role in which they are 'beaten like a rented mule'. It also raises questions around what the career path of an official is like and how it differs by sport. We address these questions in this chapter, using the latest research available. We discuss the demands of officiating, the development of skill and career trajectories. We raise topics such as motivations to become an official, what the research shows about participating in the sport you officiate, and provide examples of different factors that have had an impact on careers. Taken together, this chapter will highlight factors to consider in the development of officiating from a broader perspective, and is an excellent complement to the detail about training in Chapter 9.

The development of sports officials

To understand the best way to train for any role, whether as a police officer, an athlete or a sports official, it helps to first analyse the demands with which you are faced. How you train should be determined by what you need to train to do. In research on sports officiating it is helpful to understand that there are different roles with different demands, all under the title of sports official.

Types of officials

Three main types of officiating roles have been identified.[1, 2] These three categories of officials take into account differences in the amount of interaction with athletes and movement demands, and in the number of cues being observed. For example, a basketball referee is on the performance surface, moving about and communicating with the athletes. This is in contrast to a gymnastics judge who may have a large number of cues to track, such as the athlete's toes (pointed or flexed), rotation and positioning of multiple body parts. A tennis line judge, in comparison, is mainly concerned with watching where the tennis ball lands relative to the court lines. As Figure 2.1 shows, taking these movement and information processing factors into account, the three types of officials that have been identified are:

- *interactors* – with high interaction and physical movement demands and often a large number of cues to process, as in the soccer referee
- *sport monitors* – with low to medium interaction and physical demands, but often a medium to large number of cues to monitor, as shown in the gymnastics judge
- *reactors* – with low interaction and movement demands and a low to medium number of cues to track, as in the case of the tennis line judge described above.

There is some overlap between these categories; however, this model for classifying officials works well in distinguishing the major types. We will refer to this model throughout this book as a way of acknowledging the differences in the roles and clarifying the information we present about officials and how this information applies to the different types.

Motives for becoming a sports official (and avoiding drop out)

There are a range of motivations that officials report. Interactor officials may enjoy the physical aspect of officiating and use the activity as a means to maintain fitness. Some officials enjoy the mental side, and find knowing and understanding the rules of a sport in depth or the process of making decisions and judgements and providing

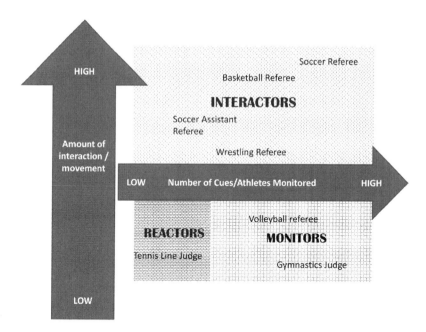

FIGURE 2.1   Categories of officials. From Plessner & MacMahon.[2]

the fairest playing environment possible appealing challenges. Some officials say that they have retired from the sport as players or athletes, perhaps due to injury, and want a way to stay involved[3] for the love of the sport.[4] Others see officiating as a way to 'give back' to their sport or as a way to serve the community. In some cases, particularly in reactor roles, officials may become involved as volunteers to support a child's participation. For example, as a track and field official, a parent can become certified by scoring 80 per cent or above in a certification test,[5] and the role may have very minimal physical demands (see Chapter 3 for more on physical demands in officials, and Chapter 9 for more on training and qualification of officials). At the early stages of involvement in officiating, salary is not a major motivator.[6] Younger officials often say that they are driven by individual factors such as developing a career.[6] Later on, however, salary has effects on performance and retention, and recognition becomes influential. For example, a 2011 study by English researchers[7] found that salaried referees, in contrast to referees paid on a match-by-match basis, showed better refereeing performance. The implication this study makes is that salary is a performance motivator that leads to superior performance at this stage. Other factors that come with professionalisation may also play a part at this stage, however, such as the fact that salaried referees may be motivated to maintain high performance standards to retain their salaried position, or that they may be required to take part in more rigorous training or have access to better training resources.

BOX 2.1 SALARIES

Salaries vary among professional officials based on sport and also seniority within sport. These variations can sometimes lead to dispute and strikes. In this sphere, some commentators also note that, when officiating salaries are 'too low', the temptation to fix games increases. Below we compare information on salaries (in US dollars) for three of the major sports in the US.

In 2012 the National Football League (NFL) ratified a new eight year contract with the referees' union. This contract, the longest referees' contract in the history of the NFL, increased salaries from $149,000 in 2011 to $173,000 in 2013. By 2019, the salary will be $205,000.[8] This followed on the heels of controversy after the league used replacement referees from lower levels of competition, including the Legends Football League (renamed in 2013, formerly the Lingerie Football League, in which female athletes compete in 7 on 7 American football, donning lingerie; clothing changed from lingerie to 'performance wear' in 2013, although there is little noticeable difference other than the absence of more obvious lingerie-like apparel such as garters). Several cases of controversial calls or errors added convincingly to the case that the NFL umpires represented an essential role within the sport, with a high level of skill in a difficult job.

In the National Basketball Association, referees reportedly earn between $100,000 and $300,000 per year. Though this has increased from between $18,146 and $78,259 in 1983, an increase of 136 per cent, player salaries, currently averaged at $5.2 million, have increased 806 per cent over the same period. In 1983 the average player salary was $275,000.[9]

Major League Baseball appears to have a large variation in salary. In 2009 the range was reported to be from $84,000 per year up to $400,000 each year, with seniority, and first class travel to games. This is in contrast to the reported salary in the minor leagues, which starts at $1,800 a month and moves only to $3,200 in triple A. At this minor league level, the salary also only applies to the three to five months in-season. The minor league salary and lack of first class travel fits with the description of this phase of participation and development as the 'hard slog' mentioned.[5]

Part of the reason why salary may be unimportant early but becomes influential later may be that, although there are attractive salaries at the highest level in some sports (see Box 2.1), the number of officials at this elite end is small, and it is often a 'hard slog' to rise up the ranks. This is illustrated by a quote from Jim Caple, a baseball journalist who, after criticising Major League umpires, wrote about his visit to an umpiring school:

> I've met some major league players who are indifferent to the game – one former player told me that when he was in the minors, he preferred losing to winning because then they didn't have to play the bottom of the ninth – but a deep love of baseball is absolutely mandatory for a pro umpire. Without it, there is no way you could endure the years of poverty-level wages, the months away from loved ones, the nights spent sharing cheap motel rooms

with a partner, the endless heckling and complaints from managers, players and fans, the constant family sacrifices.[10]

So, in the face of this 'hard slog', if it's not salary, what is the main motivator for becoming an official? Is it as simple as a deep love of the sport, as Jim Caple seems to think? A number of studies show that the motivator is not only love of the sport, as the quote above shows, but social interaction,[6] a sense of community[11] and commitment to the sport.[12] Officials indicate that a sense of connection and socialising with the athletes and other officials brings enjoyment to the role. They are also more likely to continue officiating if they have an identity as an official.[12] This gives us some good information about how to keep officials who are 'in the programme'.

Keeping the main motivators for engaging in officiating in mind, some officials have lamented that, as they become more proficient and move up the competition levels, socialising and interacting with athletes is viewed as a source of bias and is thus informally discouraged. In a similar vein, the issue of abuse of the official is critical, not only because it creates difficulty for the official or for players but because it may interfere with the connection and enjoyment that officials feel in their role, which could then lead to drop out. This is particularly critical for inexperienced and younger officials who are reportedly more likely to be abused, and experience greater stress and drop out as a result.[13–15] So, like salary, the impact of abuse on officials may depend on the level of officiating. Although some Australian researchers found no connection between abuse and drop out,[16] this was in a sample of professional and semi-professional officials. At this level, many officials have learned to reinterpret abuse as part of the role. These are the type of officials represented in the commercial we described at the beginning of the chapter: they are able to 'take it' and not react, because it is seen as a part of the job, and they have trained to cope with it. At this level, abuse is reported as an unpleasant aspect of the job. At lower levels of involvement, however, abuse is more likely to create stress and threaten participation and progression, not only because of a greater volume or amount of abuse and lesser skill for dealing with it, but also because of its interference with social connection as a more central motivator. As one research study shows,[12] stressors (such as abuse and the physical demands of the role; see Chapter 3 for more on physical demands) and commitment to the sport work in opposite ways: stressors interfere with the retention of officials and commitment and identification as an official increases likelihood to continue.

As we have alluded to, the inadvertent removal or de-emphasis of aspects of officiating that are key motivators for the individual is an important consideration in retaining officials in the role, but also to maintain and improve performance (see Chapter 9 for more discussion about recruiting and retaining officials). Increasing the connection with other officials provides social interaction and involvement with the sport, as well as reinforcing identification as an official to maintain and increase commitment. Officiating done in teams can also benefit from rapport, improved communication and cohesion.[17] This is true at all levels of performance. For example, in 2009, Steven Walkom, then director of officiating for the National

Hockey League, discussed the importance he placed on fostering cohesion within the officials at the 2009 meeting of the National Association of Sports Officials. Group-based activities like an adventure race at a country retreat and open communication were used to create a team-like approach within the officials so that assignment to officiate key games (e.g., Stanley Cup finals) was celebrated rather than envied within the group.

Career paths and levels of officiating

The classification of officials we presented earlier – interactor, monitor and reactor – considers the movement and decision demands of the specific role. It's clear that, in our previous sections, things like motivations, salary and abuse are seen differently depending on the stage or level of officiating. We think it's useful, in understanding development, to discuss these differences using a framework that comes from work with athletes. The FTEM (Foundations, Talent, Elite, Mastery) framework has been devised to describe and optimise the development pathways of athletes.[18] Although there is much less formal research on the development of officials, we have adapted the FTEM framework here (see Figure 2.2) to help illustrate the complexity of officiating development and to make the point clear that there are a number of different levels and types of officials as well as pathways that referees, judges and umpires may take. Using this framework helps to provide a way to think about optimising pathways and supporting development and reminds us about these differences in motivation, the impact of abuse and salary.

Our adaptation of the FTEM framework has avoided 'tinkering' too much for two reasons: first, because the original framework is very flexible, allowing it to be fitted to specific sports and contexts, which captures athlete pathways and development very well; and, second, because we acknowledge that the framework would be similarly adapted to specific sports and officiating structures which differ by country and even region. The major difference when we consider the development of athletes and the development of officials, however, is that we need to account for experience in both the athlete and official role, given how common it is to come to officiating from playing. This is where capturing officiating development becomes complex: some people both compete and officiate in multiple sports either sequentially or concurrently. In addition, coaching should also be considered. So we stress here that we have adapted this framework to be a very general descriptor that can be modified.

We'll first talk about the major stages of the framework (F, T, E and M) and then the pathways that can lead across to and between any of these levels (active lifestyle, sport and sport excellence).

FTEM stages and levels

The FTEM describes four main stages of participation, each with levels within them.[18] These are the foundation (3), talent (4), elite (2) and mastery (1) stages.

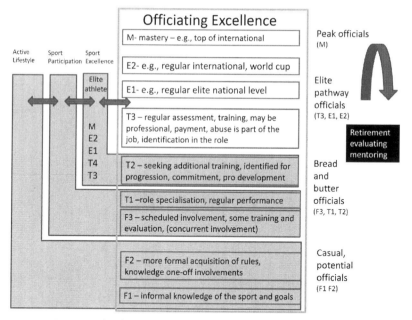

FIGURE 2.2 Framework of development for officials. Adapted from Gulbin *et al.*[18]

In officiating, the foundation stage is the general knowledge acquisition stage. This is where the basic structures and rules of a sport are learned. The first stage (F1) describes the informal casual learning that can be gained as a participant or observer (e.g., parent). For many, this basic knowledge is acquired simply due to the popularity and thus exposure to a sport, such as soccer in Brazil. This level of knowledge can be acquired with little participation, as reflected in the overlap with the active lifestyle pathway, which is discussed in more detail below.

F2 represents more structured but still core knowledge, introducing formal certification and course training. This can be accompanied by some practical experience; however, this experience is casual and often informal, represented by, for example, officiating an exhibition, practice or casual competition. F2 officials can be labelled 'occasional officials'. This stage also picks up athletes who need to be their own official, as is the case in the lower developing levels in tennis, and also coaches who are asked to fill in in the officiating role.

We use the F3 stage to help describe when individuals first start to become more attracted and committed to the role of official. This point may begin a transition from them taking on an identity as an official, although hyphenated (e.g., player-referee) at F3, to an unhyphenated official and regular involvement and assignment to competitions in a scheduled season, which is characteristic of the talent stage of development.

The talent stage is perhaps the most interesting and also critical stage for officiating. This is where regular performance begins. It can be the gateway to elite performance, to maintenance of regular participation or to drop out. The talent stage is typically where the 'hard slog' happens and where the most significant barriers are successfully or unsuccessfully negotiated. The officials at the T1 and T2 levels are regularly officiating at regional levels. They may be interested in or have been identified as those with potential to progress up the pathway. Others at the T1 and T2 levels are happy to remain engaged at this level. We refer to these individuals as 'bread and butter officials' because, while they have committed to the role, they are motivated by the love of the sport, social interaction and giving back to the community, and are happy at this level of involvement, not necessarily moving up to elite levels. Within a sport that has a large volume of games or competitions to be officiated at the lower and intermediate levels of participation, these are the folk who help the sport run from week to week and feed into the bigger system – the bread and butter of the sport.

As mentioned, many of the T1 and T2 bread and butter officials are not explicitly aiming to progress to perform at elite levels of competition. The alternative activities and commitments that they have may prevent greater investment, as described in the Sport Commitment Model.[19, 20] This model predicts participation in light of competing activities. Keep in mind that these officials may still be skilled and elite (see Box 2.2) at this level but, depending on the demands of the specific sport, and particularly with interactor roles with high physical demands, they may not be on a pathway to professional status or to officiating at the highest level of competition in the sport and dedicate fewer hours to the role.

BOX 2.2 WHAT IS EXPERTISE IN OFFICIATING?

In this chapter we show that there are a variety of officials, defined not only by demands (interactor, monitor, reactor; see Figure 2.1) but also by the context or level at which they officiate, such as the casual potential official, the bread and butter and the peak or mastery level official (see Figure 2.2). But what makes an official an *expert*? In officiating (and coaching) we often confuse the level of participation with the level of expertise of an individual; we think that officials at the elite level are experts, and those officiating athletes at lower levels are less skilled. This thinking ignores the fact that the characteristics, strengths and skills that are needed at each level are different. For example, an official working with beginning soccer players is concerned with a safe playing environment, often with educating the players about the game, and with ensuring that there is a fun environment to encourage participation and engagement. This requires skills very different from those at the elite level where physical fitness may be emphasised, each decision is subject to scrutiny and managing the emotions of players as well as coaching staff becomes key. As well, the types of calls, their frequency and the speed at which play unfolds can differ at each level, and officials become attuned to the general play, typical patterns and capabilities of players. The resources available to officials also differ, which often dictates the skills that are required. For example, at lower levels of competition the official may have more responsibility, given a lack of available line judges and timekeepers, meaning they may need to use and manage volunteers or keep time themselves.

(continued)

(continued)

The difference in demands at higher levels of play was clearly demonstrated during the 2012 NFL referee strike. During the strike the league used replacement referees. Where previously replacements came from the college level, these replacements were from recreational leagues including what was then called the Lingerie League. While the replacements may have been skilled in the context of their particular leagues and demands, many incidents showed they were not accustomed to the NFL level. A good example happened in the final play of a close game between Green Bay and Seattle, when Seattle trailed by only two points. When the ball was caught in the end zone by a Green Bay player and, after falling to the ground, was also held by a Seattle player, two officials signalled opposing calls. During this strike period there were also hefty fines to coaches who displayed frustration with officials, asking for explanations (and in the process grabbing an official's arm, in one case), or otherwise abusing the officials.[21]

Progression through the talent stage and levels may also be limited by the age at which an individual becomes involved as an official, depending on the sport. For example, although a gymnastics judge can become an official later, after a full career as an athlete, and still expect to be able to progress, this may not be the case in many interactor sports. In soccer, research has shown that it takes as long as 16 years to reach the FIFA level of officiating,[22] and most officials at this level specialised as referees in their teens. It is thus rare to specialise late and progress to elite levels in some sports. On the other hand, a retired player who is seeking to remain connected to the sport but is interested in a lesser time commitment may move into a T1 or T2 official and not be attracted to the T3 and T4 levels. The youngster looking to push through to the elite levels of involvement, also at T1 and T2, is on a different path and looking for more commitment and activities and training, which can come from T3 and T4.

With continued training, progression and motivation, the T3 and T4 officials, as per the original FTEM framework, can be labelled 'pre-elites'. These officials have strengthened commitment, increased volume of training and performance activities and, depending on the sport, some compensations for the role. They may now be travelling to perform on regional and interstate/inter-provincial levels. These officials are at the critical level where support for continued development can be tricky: the E1 and E2 levels are at the professional level where funding often supports training and evaluation resources and salary can help to ease the time commitment to the role in order to take up and participate in more training to improve performance. Officials at the T3 and T4 levels, however, are likely to be those who are in the 'hard slog' described earlier for baseball umpires, where there is a threat of dropping down to lower levels (T2, T1) or dropping out entirely. Here we should also point out that the framework is a loose and generalised descriptor, with each sport differing – there may be fewer levels or, as the authors of the FTEM for sport describe, progression through phases can be as short as months or as long as decades.

The last two stages are elite and mastery. The elite stage broadly describes the regular elites, such as the first league referee (E1), and the regular finals and championship officials from this group (E2). Starting from the end of the talent stage, these officials are at a stage in which abuse is regarded as part of the job, as mentioned before, where compensation becomes more critical, and salary disputes have an impact on the league (see Box 2.1), and where training needs may include media training and resources for complex legal issues.

At the E2 level, officials are consistently performing at the regular elite level, with a fixed recurring commitment and high level of performance. At E1 and E2 there is a clear role and time commitment. We have adapted the mastery level to describe those who have been selected from these regularly high performing elites to events such as the Olympics and World Championships. Because innovation, standing out and performances which change the sport are not hallmarks of elite performance in officials in the same way as they may be for athletes like Dick Fosbury or Tiger Woods,[23] regular performance at the pinnacle of the sport is appropriate for describing mastery officials.

We point out again that there may be fewer clear stages and levels in officiating in general, and particularly in sports with little development or distinction between stages. The elite and mastery levels may be very different in different sports – for example, an NBA paid professional official is considered at the elite level, as is an international panel squash official who still maintains a full time job outside this role.

No matter the number of stages and levels appropriate to one sport, the advantage to this model is that it helps to capture involvement from the casual one-off involvement that might happen at a junior level or an exhibition level by a parent acting as an occasional official, for example, to more regular scheduled involvement and levels in which training is undertaken, up to professionalisation and peak performance. It helps consider issues such as converting the foundation stage of knowledge and activity into the talent stage with regular involvement, and understanding drop out versus progression from this talent stage. We have touched on some differences in how individuals can move through the stages and levels of the FTEM as we have adapted it to officiating. We will now turn to discussing these different paths more directly.

The FTEM pathways: active lifestyle, sport participation, sport excellence

A key feature of the FTEM framework is that it takes into account the three different sport pathways – active lifestyle, sport participation and sporting excellence – alongside the officiating excellence pathway. This captures a variety of different types of officials (e.g., occasional, bread and butter, elite) and their pathways into and out of officiating, represented by the arrows linking horizontally between these pathways in Figure 2.2, in addition to the possibility of moving vertically, sometimes with a parallel between two pathways, or in multiple sports.

The framework can also capture periods of suspended involvement and re-entry, mostly occurring at the lower levels of the officiating excellence pathway. For example, an analysis of officials in the Canadian province of Quebec[1] showed that many officials' careers have a pattern in which they officiate, have a short layoff of a number of years perhaps due to career or family demands, and then come back to officiating the sport later. At this point they may need only a short time at a lower level of involvement before progressing up the pathway again, or may even choose to remain involved at a lower level.

In Figure 2.2 you can also see that there are features common to all pathways and those that distinguish between them. For example, all pathways go through a stage where knowledge of the sport is acquired. The sport excellence and officiating excellence pathways also share common features up to the T2 level, where they are both characterised by individuals at this stage who seek additional training, are identified for progression and show commitment and professional development. At the T3 level, however, the athlete and official become much more differentiated. This is where we previously described the role-committed unhyphenated official, and where the sport general skills shared with athletes such as goal setting, basic fitness and generic visual skills are replaced by the need for more role-specific skills for the official. These are the skills such as referee-specific positioning and communication – the skills we discuss in this book. Although officials are acquiring referee-specific skills all the way along the officiating excellence pathway, perhaps in conjunction with athlete skills, the focus becomes much more crucial at this stage, with less probability of occupying playing and officiating roles both at competitive levels.

Chris Pollock, an International Rugby Board (IRB) referee, is an example of the transition from sport participation and/or sport excellence as an athlete to sporting excellence as an official. A recurring ankle injury forced him to take a season off playing, during which he refereed as a means of still staying involved in the sport. His enjoyment of refereeing, however, saw him give up playing for this new role.[24]

This early transition for Pollock, when he may have still had competitive drive, could be a key factor to his subsequent success and ability to progress to elite levels. Although Chris's injury may be a chance event that drove his career,[25] often the change of role from athlete to official can be a strategic decision. Large talent pools in sports such as soccer create high competition among athletes. Someone who is motivated to get to the elite level of the sport may see officiating as a more viable pathway than as a competitor. There is evidence from soccer to support this idea of strategic transitions from playing to officiating, and age as a key factor. The relative age effect is where athletes born later in a selection year (e.g., a December birthdate versus a January birthdate, when the selection year starts on 1 January), who are relatively younger than their peers, are disadvantaged early on, perhaps due to being physically smaller and less developed. Later-born athletes are often underrepresented at elite levels.[26] Although the younger players may 'catch up' with their peers later, by the time they do they have missed out on opportunities and resources, like better coaching, that come with selection for more elite teams. A French study indirectly supports the idea that early recognition of limited playing prospects may lead to the transition of some athletes to refereeing. It showed that, in some referee groups, there were more later-born (relatively younger) referees. The idea is that they may have switched to the referee role early on because their age disadvantaged them as athletes but not as referees.[27]

Early specialisation in officiating, as might happen with a relatively younger soccer player, may be a priority in interactor sports, given that we know it takes a long period of time to reach the peak level, as we reviewed previously.[22] Other sports officiating roles with lower movement demands, such as baseball umpiring or volleyball refereeing which are closer to the sport monitor classification, may allow for a later specialisation in this role while still allowing for a preceding athletic career and progression to relatively elite officiating levels. This is particularly the case for sport-monitored form-based sports such as women's gymnastics or diving in which athletes peak very young. The FTEM acknowledges these differences and allows for multiple entry points. In addition, although some sports have traditionally required officials to progress through all of the levels of officiating on the pathway to elite performance, regardless of their background, some now recognise the value in multiple flexible pathways including accelerated pathways for elite athletes who want to transition into officiating. Prior experience as a competitor is recognised with an accelerated progression, performance at a higher level earlier and mentoring catered to facilitating this transition. This accelerated pathway takes advantage of assumed transfer of skills and knowledge, which we discuss in the next section.

Transfer

Accelerated pathways for developing athletes into officials raises the question whether past competitive experience in the sport is necessary for elite officiating. When we described the FTEM as adapted to officiating, there is a heavy assumption that most officials have participated in the sport they officiate. However, this framework also picks up those who do not (e.g., parents), as well as the variety of extent of involvement, from those limited to community and local club levels of participation all the way up to those who were elite, competing on the highest level, before or in conjunction with becoming officials.

At the elite levels of officiating, however, it can be rare to find a sports official who has no experience of competing in the sport they officiate. This does not mean that experience in the sport is necessarily an important factor in developing skill. It may be that officials are simply attracted to changing roles within a sport with which they are familiar. To further understand the contribution of competitive experience, a number of studies have explored this topic.

Given that players, coaches and referees have different roles within the sport and make different types of decisions, one study compared how people in these three roles process information by asking each group to perform a playing, coaching and refereeing task.[22] Although it was expected that the players would outperform the other groups in the playing task, and so on and so forth, with each role showing superiority in their role-based task, this was not the case. Instead, previous experience as a player had a lasting influence on the ability to perform the player-based task, even if coaches and referees had not been in a player role for decades. There was also no difference in the referee-specific task of identifying and naming infractions (e.g., a charge/block in basketball). Although this may have been too easy a task to tap in to referee-specific skill, and perhaps different more challenging tasks would reveal referee superiority (e.g., referee positioning), it does show that knowledge in coaching and playing can also contribute to at least some aspect of refereeing.

Two more studies focused on whether motor experience (experience performing the skills being evaluated) contributes to officiating skill. In one of these studies,[28] soccer players were given experience of 'faking' (simulating) penalties in soccer to understand whether this experience would then enhance their ability to pick up faking in a video-based decision task. They were compared with a group that watched this faking training and a group that did not either perform or watch performance of fakes. In this way, motor experience (physically learning to fake) and visual experience (watching the faking training) were compared with no training to see if performance before and after these experiences would contribute. It turns out that this training did not contribute as much to the ability to pick up deceptive actions as prior accumulated experience watching soccer.

A final study controlled the motor experience in a different way.[29] Gymnastics judges were divided into those who could and those who could not perform a particular skill on the beam. The judges who were able to perform the skill performed better when asked to judge this move than the judges who were not able to do the move. Although more work needs to be done in this area, this is a pretty striking finding, and clearly there seems to be a positive contribution from competing to evaluating motor skills, especially when one particular skill, which is a focus of evaluation, is targeted.

We do, however, acknowledge the flip side – that there may be some negative transfer from being an athlete to being an official. For example, in the early stages an athlete making the officiating transition may need to 'unlearn' player positioning and fight the tendency to move in 'following player' patterns. Overall, though, it does seem that experience in the sport contributes positively, and pathways from elite competitor to elite official can capitalise on this finding. So, to answer our question, it may not be *necessary* to have experience competing in the sport one is officiating but it helps, particularly to progress to elite levels, and this is recognised by accelerated pathways. One final point with regard to transfer is that it also goes the other way: experience as an official can be beneficial for other areas of functioning (see Box 2.3), which can be a positive by-product of recent strategies in recruitment of officials.

> ## BOX 2.3 TRAINING AND RECRUITMENT OF OFFICIALS FROM NON-TRADITIONAL SOURCES
>
> In recent years, many sports have needed to emphasise recruiting and training officials in order to bolster dwindling numbers and participation rates. This has led to some more innovative and creative efforts in a number of sports. For example, Major League Baseball (MLB) has recently adopted a scouting approach similar to that used when recruiting athletes. The MLB's Urban Youth Academies have long provided baseball playing instruction around the country (and in Puerto Rico). Officiating has now been included as a potential pathway, not only for the 8–17-year-olds but for former players, current officials and the relatively novice, including former Marine 'students'. One-day camps are used to recruit and bring novices into the system. Recruits may progress from one-day testing to week-long training and possible scholarships to five-week umpire training schools that can lead to qualification as minor league umpires, on the path to the major leagues. This strategy helps to identify potential officials earlier and shortcut the pathway up to elite levels, as described in Figure 2.2, by providing a greater volume of structured training for a larger number of individuals.[30]
>
> Australian Rules Football has also used more novel methods to increase the number of officials participating. One of these strategies has been the creation of programmes to train and employ minimum security prison inmates. Programmes have been run across the country in Tasmania, Victoria and the Northern Territory, particularly in remote areas where the viability of competitions was threatened due to umpire shortages. These programmes not only increase the numbers in the ranks of officials, a welcome outcome, but also provide benefits to the participants where on-field skills transfer to life off-field. As Tasmanian Umpiring manager Michael Brown commented about the Tasmanian programme: "Through this program they learn discipline, co-ordination, decision making and the need to display fairness – all essential attributes for a constructive role back in the community".[31,32]

Retirement

If we are discussing development of sports officiating, we should also discuss the end – when one is no longer an official. Australian researchers report that most sports officials quit within five years after becoming accredited.[13] Thus, many sports organisations have shifted their emphasis from recruitment to recruitment *and* retention, which is addressed in more detail in Chapter 9. This is also relevant for the many officials who follow the pattern we have discussed of having a 'lay off' for a number of years and then returning to the sport. Again, in this case, officials may 'begin again' at a different level of the officiating excellence pathway. They may then progress rapidly through the levels as they regain and refine their skills.

Quitting is different from retiring, however. Quitting officiating implies issues with commitment; either lack of commitment to the role or competition from other commitments. In comparison, retirement implies that a career or involvement has come to an end, often because of declining abilities. Retirement may occur in greater numbers for the bread and butter (F3, T1, T2), elite (T3, E1, E2) or peak (M) official role. Again we see that the demands of the different officiating types play a role in considerations for retirement. For the sport monitor and the reactor, where the major demands are perceptual-cognitive, performance may be less hampered by declining physical abilities and things like speed, which are concerns for the interactor official such as the soccer referee. Regardless of the specific type of skill or ability that suffers a decline, however, it is important to acknowledge that individuals decline at different rates and that, often, cognitive skills such as knowing where to be can help compensate for a loss of physical skills and fitness. The use of mandatory retirement ages is thus often somewhat arbitrary and risks missing out on individual differences. This is particularly important given that the development of an interactor official to the elite level can be lengthy; it is a shame to miss out on an individual's skills, which might in fact be at their peak, if there is no evidence of decline, simply because of an arbitrary age cut-off.

Regardless of when and why an official retires, retaining well-performing experienced officials as mentors or evaluators then becomes a focus. This is where mentors are used to train others or teach soft skills such as the best cues to use and how to interact with athletes. Although many sports have referee coaches – who may not have any experience as an official themselves – who coach more generic or fitness skills, the sport-specific experience-based skills that a retired official has are invaluable, particularly to those at the crucial transition stages. Development in the elite officiating pathway should thus also consider when an individual moves to the mentor stage, after retirement. Of course, it is helpful to remember that not every good performer is a good mentor. This is similar to the accepted knowledge that not every elite athlete makes a good coach. But, with appropriate training in teaching methods and mentoring skills, the likelihood of creating an invaluable training 'tool' from a formerly active official is increased. In this way, therefore, the pathway can feed back into itself (retired officials can also move into administration roles, feeding back into a sport in yet another role).

Injury

We used the example of Chris Pollock whose injury as an athlete was a catalyst or chance event in becoming an official. Particularly for interactor officials, injury can have a significant impact on development and performance. There isn't a great deal of research on injury in officiating, however. Most of what we know concentrates on rates and types of injury and has been collected in soccer. For example, in a sample of elite soccer referees, a 2011 English study reported that only 13 per cent of injuries occurred during performance (refereeing) and the majority (60 per cent) came from physical training.[32] When the number of injuries relative to amount of time spent in activities was considered, however, physical testing resulted in the greatest number of injuries. The fact that these tests take place in the preseason may have been a factor. At this stage, officials may still be building match levels of fitness.

A study of Irish elite referees showed a different pattern, with greater rates of injury in match officiating (16.4 injuries per 1,000 hours) compared to rates for training (8.8 per 1,000 hours).[34] This study also found that injury rates in soccer officials are higher than in other non-contact sports, and that the incidence rate of injury from training for soccer referees is higher than that of injury rates from training for soccer players. One factor that may influence this pattern is resources – in training, medical staff, equipment and times – that are available to referees in comparison to players.

The picture with regard to when injuries occur is slightly different when considering not just elites but all levels of participation. When all levels of participation were considered in a study of Swiss referees, the number of injuries from training was lower than from matches.[35] Thus, the authors recommend preventive programmes for injury. Of course, finding fewer training-related injuries in this bigger mixed-level group might be because there was less training overall compared with the elite groups in the previous studies.

The type of injuries the research uncovers seems to reflect a few factors: the demands of the officiating roles and also the general characteristics of the officials as a group. For example, injuries in the English study were mostly strains (78 per cent) and sprains (14 per cent) and, in rare cases, fractures (six per cent). The Irish study similarly found that muscle strain was the most common type of injury, the lower leg the most common site, and overuse the most cited cause. Although leg injuries in soccer are a commonality between referees and players, there are differences that are probably due to the fact that they do different things. For example, referees do not report as many knee and thigh injuries as players, which has been explained by the fact that they don't generally contact the ball or other players.[34] Another interesting difference is that the rate of Achilles injuries is higher in referees, which is attributed to their advanced age relative to players and the fact that Achilles tendon injuries are degenerative in nature, as well as the fact that referees do more backwards running than players, which puts more strain on the Achilles.[34]

One factor that may play a part in injury in officials in general is that officials have traditionally had much less of a 'culture of practice' compared with athletes. Also, as mentioned earlier, training resources, even at elite levels, are often limited. Without appropriate or adequate guidance and support, fitness testing and fitness training can indeed be a source of injury rather than the prevention of injury. More research in this area can be used to investigate these factors and lead to information on best practice.

Summary and conclusion

Let's come back to our NFL umpire, being yelled at by a coach, with the announcers asking "Where do you train to take a beating like that?" This scenario focuses on only one of a number of skills that officials must have. These skills are covered in more depth in the chapters that follow in this book. At a broad level, however, we have shown that the development of officials and how they train must consider a number of key interrelated topics:

- what motivates the official to become and remain an official
- when officials might leave and subsequently come back to participation
- the different types of officials, not only in terms of demands (interactors, monitors, reactors) but also in terms of levels of performance and goals (casual/potential, bread and butter, elite pathway, peak/mastery)
- the impact of transfer of skills from other roles on training and progression (as well as the benefit of officiating to other parts of life and professions)
- retirement from officiating and transitioning to other roles along the pathway of participation
- the impact, types and sources of injury.

What all of this shows is the complexity and the multiple possibilities in training and career progressions. We have begun to bring many of these themes together by adapting the FTEM framework to officials, and providing an approach to continue to explore questions about development.

Official's call

Janie Frampton

Referees have to be passionate and committed and the rest will fall into place, as then they are more likely to undertake the learning and development that they need to get them there. You have to be committed to your learning and not expect someone else to spoonfeed you. For soccer referees at the top level, they'll have bespoke physical training programmes to complete, which will change on a weekly basis, based on GPS and heart rate data and guidance from a sport scientist. It's difficult to expect the same sort of commitment from unpaid (non-full-time officials) as many, even those involved in Olympic sports, have to pay their own way, although many sports provide expenses or a daily rate.

The love of the sport comes first. That's what drives you. Being involved in the game on a regular basis is what officiating provides. If you know you're not the best player then, just from a statistical perspective, you've a better chance of getting to Wembley as an official. It worked in my case. The motivation from social interaction is an individual thing. It's a very insular role being a referee. Some like it and some crave the social rewards that often are needed to offset the on-field isolation. I love the fact that I feel part of a big worldwide family of refereeing.

My experience, and the limited research undertaken, suggests that women feel valued and supported through the wider social connections that refereeing brings and therefore they will be retained longer, whereas research shows the social side is not a key area for the retention of men in the same way. There are generally fewer social connections going on with the men. Women, however, will form social groups and closed Facebook sites to share their experiences. For example, we have around 1,000 women referees of which over 300 are members of a closed Facebook site where they support each other, and it helps as a great retention tool and to build that feeling of belonging. Men, on the other hand, seem to be far more individual in their role as a referee. For example, in England we have approximately 28,000 referees of whom around 27,000 are men, yet there are only approximately 7,000 members of the Referees Association in total (many of whom are retired and are therefore not counted within the 27,000, and some are female). The monthly Referee Society meetings provide a degree of interaction so, in a small way, they help to develop a sense of team building and belonging. The low membership from our masses clearly shows that men either don't need that type of social environment or there isn't one that they feel fits their needs.

Refereeing can be a big commitment. At the top end from level 4 (supply league) to level 1 (national list), soccer referees have regular body mass index, body fat and weight measurements taken – so they have to reach levels similar to those of elite athletes. These things are important but, if you have six per cent body fat, which may be better than the levels of elite athletes, does it make you a better referee? Sometimes too much is placed on this. Image, of course, is very important, and an 'overhang' at the waistline can be a problem for the perception of others. For example, one of our top English Premiership referees recently lost two stone (nearly 30 pounds) over the summer. It doesn't make him a better referee but the perception may be that he is. I think we've got to keep these sorts of things in perspective, but also recognise that our refereeing population is not the same as the players. They tend to be older and often are carrying long-term injuries that have to be managed.

My life has been transformed by my officiating, but equally my officiating has been transformed by my life. I think probably the most important aspect of my life that has influenced my refereeing has been having children and being a parent. You learn some strong disciplines. So, if you say to your kids "If you do that again you're going to bed" and then they do it again, you have to send them to their room. Similarly, if you speak to a player who is pushing the limits and you warn them, you have to be true to your word. For your own credibility, if they intervene again you have to sanction them. Some referees use the staircase approach: (i) you have the quiet word, (ii) then the more obvious word, and (iii) then you begin sanctions as necessary. So, for me, parenting has been a big influence on player management.

But there are many other influences too. Playing and coaching have had a massive influence on me. I don't advocate that you have to have played or coached at any level, but the mere experience of those disciplines help your understanding of the game – and that knowledge of the game is crucial. Sometimes you need to have empathy for the coach or the player in certain situations – and it definitely helped me, having been there as a player and a coach.

My path into refereeing is probably like many others. I guess for years I stood on touchlines shouting at referees thinking I knew best – like many of us watching games today. Then my son started taking an interest in soccer. I then helped to form a youth section of our local senior club and there were never referees to officiate their games – the parents didn't even want to do it, so I said I'd take a referee's course to support youth soccer. Once I'd done the course I was very driven. I wanted to do the big boys – I wanted to do all of it. And then once I got into it and started to develop, I thought the only way I would be taken seriously was to work towards the two promotions that would take me to Senior County level. I thought then people would take me seriously. I never really had any ambition beyond that.

There were many rewards along the way, but also many challenges. You've got to be mentally tough to deal with outspoken players at times, but I think it's important not to overstate the prevalence of abuse towards referees. Even one case of abuse is too much – it's important to lead on that. But it actually happens so seldom when you consider 32,000 games of soccer are played in England every weekend. Yes, any abuse is too much – we know that, but we should be promoting all the good things about refereeing and we don't do enough of that. I guess I must have refereed over 2,000 games and there were only two in which I received abuse with which I felt uncomfortable. Other abuse you take with a pinch of salt as the passion of the moment. Still, in those early days as a female referee I perhaps took too much because we (the female officials) wanted to be accepted as referees and not as women. It's a question Wendy Toms (the first woman to come through to referee the professional game in England and also the first woman to work as a Premiership assistant referee) and I ask ourselves regularly. Did we set our tolerance level too high? Maybe we could have done more for women to be accepted more easily now – I don't know. It's tough to understand or measure. We did what we thought was right at the time by not making a fuss and taking perhaps more abuse than we should have because we wanted to be accepted. Maybe we could have changed the perception of women's refereeing if we had been a little tougher, but I don't think we'll ever really know for sure.

The driver for me and for most referees I've encountered has always been a love of the game. I was not motivated by money, and I'm not surprised that the research suggests that salary only really becomes influential later in referees' careers because of the commitment that they have to give. If you're a family person and this time is taken away from you, you need some form of payback. If that comes in being able to provide more (perhaps in monetary affordances) for your family when you *are* there, then that seems a bit fairer. However, if you're at the semi-professional level where the money is not very encouraging yet the demands on your time and commitment are almost to the level of those at the very top, then there's very little payback. At that level (3 and 4) I think it can lead to retention issues where people cannot give the time to do what they have to do and what is expected of them – things like the physical training, travel, attendance at meetings etc. I guess I'm also not surprised that salaried referees perform better than those who just receive a match fee. I think the biggest factor is probably that, when referees receive a salary, it simplifies their lives. As you progress as a referee you often have to balance a full-time job, family commitments (often kids) and, of course, the physical training and then games at the weekend and sometimes midweek. All that is a huge commitment. If you take the bulk of that time away with a nine to five job, then it takes away a huge part of your development. It would be crazy if we couldn't make officials better by bringing a bit of balance and preparation time to their busy world.

Foundation, talent, elite and mastery (FTEM) framework

I would say that the *foundation* level includes any officiating up to county level (levels 5, 6 and 7). If you can referee at county level then you can referee anywhere – that's your apprentice. It's your intra-county soccer. You are on a massive learning curve yourself as you build your knowledge, application and confidence. Anticipation of play is difficult because the game is less predictable.

When you get to level 4 (the first level of semi-professional soccer), it includes more travelling (and a greater expectation from a time perspective) – that's when it starts to get serious because your career is now managed by the Football Association and not by the county. You have to travel further and the commitment increases. The standard of everything is much higher – the commitment, the game – and we lose a lot of referees. You have to train for fitness tests and training days, which also add to the travel, and there's not so much more money but probably at least three times as much commitment. This is the start of the *talent* level. At level 4 there are probably 1,000 referees, and at level 3 probably 450. This is where you start to whittle out the talent with age and commitment. From level 4 the next level is 3, which is the higher end of semi-professional soccer. You may well have a coach at this level and again the time commitment increases, as do the number of games you cover and the distances travelled. I would say the *elite* is the first level of professional soccer from 2a (National Conference level) to level 1, which is your national list. Beyond that you're looking at the *mastery* level, who are the FIFA referees, of whom there are about seven in the English Premiership, and this places them in a group of around 100 of the top officials in Europe out of approximately 540,000 active referees across the whole of Europe (operating at the equivalent of levels 1 down to 8).

Within the elite and mastery levels the Premiership referees get marked on their games by 'delegates', who are often former players, coaches or managers who work for the PFA and they judge the referee's game from an impartial perspective, but hopefully with some empathy and understanding of the playing and coaching environment. So they'll grade everything other than their technical ability as an official. Thus, they are servicing the game from a coach/player/manager perspective rather than with a focus on helping the referee get better by looking at his positioning, etc. These guys provide really helpful information. It's still quite subjective but usually very good.

The Premiership referees will also get a decision-making mark from one assessor who will also identify Key Match Incidents (KMIs) which can then be referred to a panel (usually comprising three ex-Premier League referees) if the decision is not obvious. The referees seem to like the system because they consider it to be fair as it allows them the chance to get further reviews of incidents. I think we still often find it difficult to really capture the feeling and the tempo of the game, which can affect things, but we do factor in the level of difficulty. So, for example, if a penalty is considered wrong which might lead to a low mark, they will also be judged on the level of difficulty of that decision, which seems to balance things out a little, so again the referees consider this to be pretty fair.

The FTEM model seems to fit refereeing nicely, although sometimes I'm not sure we get the rewards and breakthroughs that we should. The appointments tend to be our reward structure – so progressing officials through the ranks. Unfortunately, sometimes the politics get in the way and we miss talent or referees have great games in one league but underperform in another and miss the cut as a consequence. Also, sometimes the good, developing officials are not rewarded because, unfortunately, again personal preference of the decision makers and politics can get in the way as well as the personal circumstances of individuals. At the semi-professional level over 60 per cent of games are covered by an assessor. In addition, at levels 3 to 7 both club secretaries mark the referee. Unfortunately, often they may not have been able to watch the game so the coach might say "He did alright but he gave a penalty in the 70th minute which was wrong – give him 40", which makes the whole marking system very subjective, especially as 'rogue marks' that have been awarded due to an unfair opinion of a club secretary stay within the merit table of the referee and reflect on the chance of promotion or relegation. We know the assessment system is not perfect, but it is better to use these marks from the assessors as the first measurement rather than the subjective view of club marks. So, when there is an assessor, he or she will mark you on a range of factors: (i) application of the law; (ii) match control; (iii) positioning, fitness and work rate; (iv) alertness and awareness (including management of stoppages); (v) communication; (vi) teamwork; and (vii) advantage. These will all be graded out of five and applied to a weighted formula (e.g., match control is multiplied by five and advantage is multiplied by two) to provide a score out of a hundred. The assessor will also write a descriptive paragraph on each of the seven areas and finally provide ideas for development and areas of strength.

At the Premiership level the officials are assessed via DVD. An assessor will have a list of timings from minute one to ninety where the assessor will enter decisions or discussion points where appropriate throughout the timings. Once entered, these points will show as either a green box for a correct decision and a red one for an incorrect decision. Then the referee will have to go through every comment, particularly the red boxes. So, for example, I looked at one of the Premiership referees recently and in one of the green boxes he wrote something like "I agree, thanks for the praise – pleased you supported me on this". On one of the red boxes he commented, " . . . from my position I was unable to see the infringement you refer to" or "I agree I missed the clear handball". The assessors get quite a lot of training on the online system and most of them have refereed to a high level, so they have a good idea of what to look for, but sometimes it's hard to get the assessor to 'feel the heat of the kitchen'. Unless you've walked in those shoes, it's sometimes very hard to understand why certain decisions are or are not given. Once you get to level 1 and 2 (in England, the Premiership, Championship and the Football League divisions 1 and 2), I think it becomes hard for the assessors. I believe up to level 3 you can develop assessors through appropriate education but, beyond level 3, I believe you have to have operated at the level you are assessing so you understand and feel the pressure, the demands and the environment. Many share my view, although others still believe you can develop people to all levels through education.

Entering and exiting the referee pathway

I can't think of any examples of direct entry to officiating at the elite or mastery level. There has been some discussion about fast tracking players. They come with an abundance of knowledge and experiences – but there's no money in it and who says they have the array of other skills that referees need? I can only think of one situation where a soccer player made it to referee at the top level. He played at Football League level and officiated at the same level, but in this particular case it didn't really work as he wasn't ever sure on which side of the fence he sat – on the players' side or in his role as a referee. On the other side of the coin, I think it's absolutely possible to referee without extensive playing experience. You don't have to have been a player. Sure it helps you to have a tactical understanding – you need to know why when they're making substitutions, and what they are trying to achieve through their game plan, but often you can get this experience from watching games. I think watching soccer is one of the most important ways of learning. We can learn from the good and the bad decisions made, and the reactions of players and managers. Exposure to all these types of situations can help a referee in his or her own game and learning how to manage situations that might arise.

Naturally, we get referees dropping out of officiating at all stages. Often the reason for referees dropping out of officiating as they progress through the FTEM model is because of the time commitment required and the shift in work/life balance that increases the demands upon them. There was a survey sent to approximately 10,000 soccer referees, and the 2,500 referees who responded suggested that many referees were policemen and accountants and the third most frequent occupation was teachers. Most of our referees in the UK are aged between 42 and 50, and the survey suggested that the reason for dropout was time, age or just the body giving up. When referees get to retirement, some of them become assessors. There's not, strictly speaking, a retirement route. Ideally you'd like to find a role for them in the development of referees as you don't want to waste that expertise, but often there's simply not a position available. We have mentors at levels 4, 5, 6 and 7. At level 4, part of their role is to identify talent for level 3. A cohort of referees at level 3 and all those above have a coach who himself would have between five and ten referees for whom he may be responsible.

European employment laws suggest that you cannot put an age cap on when referees must retire. However, I think there's a natural age where you lose your sharpness. It is suggested that, for some referees, at around 48 you are may not be as alert as you could be or fitness may be an issue. I just think that's the most natural time to finish. I do think that they should have a route out of refereeing into some other supportive role, and you also have to look at the progression of the young guys. I think there is a natural succession issue that arises with the more 'over age' referees you keep throughout the levels. This creates less opportunity for younger referees to come through as there are a limited number of places at each level, therefore potentially stopping referee development. Finding the right time to step aside for themselves and for the game is therefore a challenge. An average age of 35 for Premiership referees is too old.

The research on exposing referees to video clips of levels of simulation to develop better perceptions of player deception is fascinating. I think 'simulation' in soccer is one of the hardest points to get right. Aerial challenges and simulation are very similar in terms of the thought processes. You really have to think, first, whether the player is cheating because, in an aerial challenge, you have to decide if the player has used his arms as a 'tool' to help him jump or as a 'weapon' to stop the opponent from getting to the ball. So you need to look at where the arms are and how they are being used. Similarly, you have to look at intention when you consider simulation, which is defined as trying to deceive the referee. Interestingly, the laws don't comment upon whether there has been contact or not – it's about deception. You can be contacted, then roll over three times, and you've attempted to deceive the referee. Have they fallen as a result of the contact? Have they fallen necessarily or unnecessarily, with or without flair? Often you could say that, if the player takes off with two feet, then he's not been contacted because he's thought about it, and you simply don't have that time if it has occurred naturally. If a player falls down in a pile like a 'sack of spuds', then the chances are that the player has been contacted. These are often good indicators. Also, the reaction of team mates is often a good indicator. The surrounding players might help. You might also think you have clearly seen it and your assistant referee might have a better view. Even if they are further away, they might have a better angle.

As referees we are constantly aware of our fitness levels. I'm not surprised that a number of injuries occur during fitness testing, but also many occur in training for the tests. Referees may not be doing the right sort of training. They may well be completing their training programme, but are the programmes right for them? How well are they warming up, eating and hydrating? Many of them have 'knackered' bodies through years of completing and preparing for bleep (fitness) tests. I'm not sure we know enough yet about the damage we've done in the past with the training that we did. We may have over-trained our referees. I know that I trained a lot, but I know now that it was the wrong type of training. I used to just run, so that I could do 2,700 metres in 12 minutes (the Cooper Test), and then I knew I could do it. Nowadays there's much more cross training, circuit training, fartlek training and more variety, all of which can be more helpful. I train much more effectively now than I did back then. Nowadays, referees who progress to level 1 will get personalised training programmes, and this makes a big difference.

References

[1] MacMahon, C., & Plessner, H. (2008). The sports official in research and practice. In D. Farrow, J. Baker, and C. MacMahon (Eds). *Developing sport expertise: Researchers and coaches put theory into practice* (pp. 172–192). London: Routledge.

[2] Plessner, H., & MacMahon, C. (2013). The sport official in research and practice. In D. Farrow, J. Baker, and C. MacMahon (Eds). *Developing sport expertise: Researchers and coaches put theory into practice, 2nd Edition* (pp. 71–95). London: Routledge.

[3] Titlebaum, J. P., Haberlin, N., & Titlebaum, G. (2009). Recruitment and rentention of sports officials. *Recreational Sports Journal, 33*, 102–8.

[4] Auger, D., Fortier, J., Thibault, A., Magny, D., & Gravelle, F. (2010). Characteristics and motivations of sports officials in the province of Québec. *International Journal of Sport Management, Recreation and Tourism, 5*, 29–50.

[5] National Officials Committee of USA Track and Field. (2011). https://www.usatf.org/groups/Officials/files/certification/2013–2016/Certification-Level-Transition-Plan-2011–1C.pdf (accessed 16 March 2013).

[6] Dorsch, K. D., Riemer, H. A., Lawrence, D., Schinke, R. J., & Paskevich, D. M. (2002). The relationship between the extent and intensity of stressful experiences of Canadian minor hockey officials. http://www.sirc.ca/research_awards/documents/dorsch.pdf (accessed 16 March 2013).

[7] Bryson, A., Buraimo, B., & Simmons, R. (2011). Do salaries improve worker performance? *Labour Economics, 18*, 424–33.

[8] Martineze, M. (2012). *Referees union formally ratify contract with NFL.* Cable News Network. http://edition.cnn.com/2012/09/29/sport/football/nfl-referees-contract (accessed 16 March 2013).

[9] Rovell, D. (2007). *NBA Refs: Pay Raise May Help Integrity of Game.* Consumer News and Business Channel. http://www.cnbc.com/id/19876494 (accessed 16 March 2013).

[10] Caple, J. (2011). *Humbled by umpire school.* Entertainment and Sports Programming Network. http://sports.espn.go.com/mlb/columns/story?columnist=caple_jim&id=6161420 (accessed 5 March 2013).

[11] Kellett, P., & Warner, S. (2011). Creating communities that lead to retention: The social worlds and communities of umpires. *European Sport Management Quarterly, 11*, 471–94.

[12] Cuskelly, G., & Hoye, R. (2013). Sports officials' intention to continue. *Sport Management Review, 16*, 451–64.

[13] Cuskelly, G., & Hoye, R. (2004). *Problems and issues in the recruitment and retention of sports officials.* A report prepared for the Australian Sports Commission, Brisbane, Australia: Griffith University.

[14] Folkesson, P., Nyberg, C., Archer, T., & Norlander, T. (2002). Soccer referees' experience of threat and aggression: Effects of age, experience, and life orientation on outcome of coping strategy. *Aggressive Behavior, 28*, 317–27.

[15] Kaissidis, A., & Anshel, M. (1993). Sources and intensity of acute stress in adolescent and adult Australian basketball referees: A preliminary study. *Australian Journal of Science and Medicine in Sport, 25*, 97–103.

[16] Kellett, P., & Shilbury, D. (2007). Umpire participation: is abuse really the issue? *Sport Management Review, 10*, 209–29.

[17] Evans, C. R., & Dion, K. L. (2012). Group cohesion and performance: A meta-analysis. *Small Group Research, 43*, 690–701.

[18] Gulbin, J. P., Croser, M. J., Morley, E. J., & Weissensteiner, J. R. (2013). An integrated framework for the optimisation of sport and athlete development: A practitioner approach. *Journal of sports sciences, 31*(12), 1319–1331.

[19] Scanlan, T. K., Carpenter, P. J., Schmidt, G. W., Simons, J. P., & Keeler, B. (1993). An introduction to the Sport Commitment Model. *Journal of Sport and Exercise Psychology*, *15*, 1–15.

[20] Scanlan, T. K., Simons, J. P., Carpenter, P. J., Schmidt, G. W., & Keeler, B. (1993). The Sport Commitment Model: Measurement development for the youth-sport domain. *Journal of Sport and Exercise* Psychology, *15*, 16–38.

[21] Wilner, B. (2012). *NFL referee strike ends*. MPRnews. http://www.mprnews.org/story/2012/09/27/daily-circuit-nfl-referees (accessed 13 March 2013).

[22] MacMahon, C., Helsen, W. F., Starkes, J. L., & Weston, M. (2007). Decision-making skills and deliberate practice in elite association football referees. *Journal of Sports Sciences*, *25*, 65–78.

[23] Starkes, J. L, Cullen, J., & MacMahon, C. (2004). A model of skill acquisition and retention of perceptual-motor performance. In A. M. Williams & N. J. Hodges (Eds). *Skill acquisition in sport: Research, theory and practice* (pp. 259–81). London: Routledge.

[24] Sports New Zealand. (2013). *Sports coaches/officials coach and instruct athletes, and officiate at sporting events.* CareerNZ. http://www.careers.govt.nz/jobs/sport-and-recreation/sports-coachofficial/about-the-job (accessed 24 February 2014).

[25] Gagné, F. (2004). Transforming gifts into talents: the DMGT as a developmental theory 1. *High Ability Studies*, *15*, 119–47.

[26] Baker, J., Schorer, J., & Cobley, S. (2010). Relative age effects. *Sportwissenschaft*, *40*, 26–30.

[27] Delorme, N., Radel, R., & Raspaud, M. (2013). Relative age effect and soccer refereeing: A 'Strategic Adaptation' of relatively younger children? *European Journal of Sport Science*, *13*, 400–6.

[28] Pizzera, A., & Raab, M. (2012). Does motor or visual experience enhance the detection of deceptive movements in football? *International Journal of Sports Science and Coaching*, *7*, 269–84.

[29] Pizzera, A. (2012).Gymnastic judges benefit from their own motor experience as gymnasts. *Research Quarterly for Exercise and Sport*, *83*, 603–7.

[30] Fordin, S. (2013). *A grass-roots approach to finding tomorrow's umps*. Major League Baseball. http://mlb.mlb.com/news/article.jsp?ymd=20130223&content_id=41930042&vkey=news_mlb&c_id=mlb_(accessed 13 March 2013).

[31] Henderson A. (2010). *Alice Springs inmates fill AFL ref shortage*. Australian Broadcasting Corporation. http://www.abc.net.au/am/content/2010/s2869220.htm (accessed 13 March 2013).

[32] Henderson, A. (2010). *Praise for prisons to footy refs program*. Australian Broadcasting Corporation. http://www.abc.net.au/news/stories/2010/04/10/2869276.htm?site=alice springs (accessed 13 March 2013).

[33] Paes, M. R., Fernandez, R., & Da Silva, A. I. (2011). Injuries to football (soccer) referees during matches, training and physical tests: original research article. *International Sports Medicine Journal*, *12*, 74–84.

[34] Wilson, F., Byrne, A., & Gissane, C. (2011). A prospective study of injury and activity profile in elite soccer referees and assistant referees. *Irish Medical Journal*, *104*, 295–7.

[35] Bizzini, M., Junge, A., Bahr, R., & Dvorak, J. (2011). Injuries of football referees: a representative survey of Swiss referees officiating at all levels of play. *Scandinavian Journal of Medicine and Science in Sports*, *21*, 42–7.

3
PHYSICAL DEMANDS

Introduction

Depending on the type of sports officiating, different physical demands are put on sports officials to successfully fulfil their job. Interactors such as soccer and basketball referees need to consistently keep up with play, positioning themselves near the centre of play in order to have optimal viewing perspectives (see Figure 3.1). This requires a number of physical demands that will be described and summarised in this chapter. This chapter will illustrate which criteria are used to measure and evaluate physical fitness of sports officials and show how and why they differ from each other.

Several studies exist that examine the physical demands of sports officials. However, these differ significantly concerning the physical aspects that have been measured. Researchers have attempted to compare and provide overviews of the different physical demands of varying sports. A good structure to sum up the findings is provided by Reilly and Gregson[1] as well as by Castagna, Abt and D'Ottavio.[2] Both distinguish between activities of soccer referees during match play and physiological responses to these activities. Castagna, Abt and D'Ottavio[2] additionally define a third category: physical capacities of referees. Although both articles focus on soccer referees, this categorisation can also be applied to other sports involving interactors (see Table 3.1 for an overview).

Activities during match play

Sports officials have to cover great distances during games in order to keep up with the play. Researchers have attempted to measure these distances using different

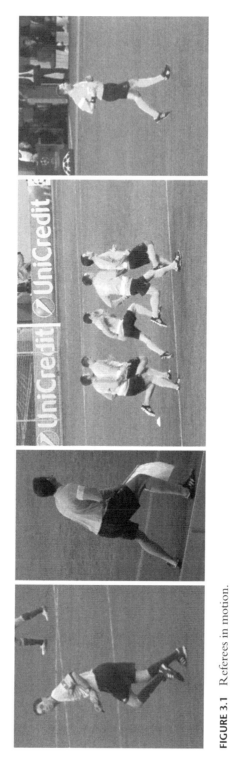

FIGURE 3.1 Referees in motion.

TABLE 3.1 Physical demands of sports officiating[2]

| Physical demands of sports officiating | | |
Activities during match play	Physiological responses	Physical capacities
Distance covered	Heart rate	Anthropometry
Match activities	Aerobic involvement	Maximal oxygen uptake
Match activities profiles	Blood lactate	Anaerobic performance
Work–rest ratios	Hydration status	Fitness testing

match analysis methods, such as detailed video analyses. The referee's stride lengths and numbers of strides are measured using on-field marking as references. Different locomotive categories are determined for this motion analysis, such as walking, jogging, low-speed running, moderate-speed running, high-speed running, sprinting, running sideways and backwards. For each category the mean speed is determined after detailed studies of videotapes. For each activity the frequency and duration are recorded and then presented for different intervals. In order to estimate the distance, the product of total time and mean speed for each activity is calculated (see Figure 3.2 for an example of the sequential process of distance estimation).[3]

Another method of measuring physical distances covered by referees is the so-called 'bi-dimensional photogrammetic system' based on direct linear transformation algorithms, which was originally used to analyse soccer players by means of a digitisation process.[4] This method also uses video-taped games for analyses, with side lines of known lengths for calibration purposes. A specific software (Photo23D) then allows digitisation of players or referees[5] at a frequency of 2 Hz, resulting in *xy* coordinates of the position to measure distances covered. More recently, the use of Global Positioning System (GPS) technology has also been applied to refereeing research.[6] A GPS transmitter is directly attached to the referee's body, collecting and storing positional data at a sampling frequency of 1 Hz.

Most studies involving the measurement of distances covered examine soccer referees. The fact that the game of soccer has changed remarkably in the past few years – in that it is faster and players are fitter – is reflected in the increased focus on fitness training for referees. However, studies which could provide a basis for training show fluctuations in distances measured (for an overview see Table 3.2).

The reasons for these fluctuations lie in the different match analysis methods (see above), categorisation of locomotive activities as well as different skill level, role (referee, assistant referee) and number of observations. Researchers have also examined referees of different countries and league levels, several seasons or only one season. However, in sum, a mean of about 10 km of distance covered by referees can be observed, which is comparable to a midfield player who generally covers the whole field as opposed to a defensive or offensive player. For an overview of distances covered by assistant referees, see Mallo, et al.[17] Other sports have also examined distances covered by referees, such as rugby,[18, 19] measuring distances of 6.7 km and 8.6 km, respectively, and 5.9 km in futsal.[20] Basketball

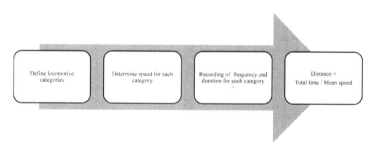

FIGURE 3.2 Sequential process of distance estimation.

referees have been shown to cover 4–6 km per match, with distances increasing throughout competition phases from qualifying to the final.[21] Nevertheless, studies in other sports remain scarce.

Since players consistently change game velocities as well as playing directions, referees are repeatedly challenged to adapt their match activities. This involves switching between standing still, running at different velocities, and backwards or sideways running. Studies have revealed that referees change their exercise modes at least 1,268 times during one competitive match play.[16] Referees spend most of the 90 minutes standing and walking, followed by jogging, running and sprinting (see Table 3.3 for an overview of studies).

From these data, work–rest ratios can be estimated, providing concrete and accurate activity profiles of referees. Both aerobic and anaerobic energy systems need to be taken into account. This information is crucial for fitness training for referees as it shows that programmes involving several jogging sessions per week are not sufficient. On the contrary, fitness programmes should focus on different exercise modes as well as endurance in order to mimic the physical demands of a competitive match as closely as possible (see Box 3.1 for physical training and testing by FIFA).

TABLE 3.2 Overview of studies estimating distance covered by soccer referees

Authors	Publication year	Distance covered
Barbero-Alvarez, et al.[7]	2012	10.2 km
Weston, Drust, & Gregson[8]	2011	11.3 km
Weston, et al.[9]	2011	11.8 km
Weston, et al.[10]	2010	11.5 km
Krustrup, et al.[3]	2009	10.3 km
Da Silva, Fernandes, & Fernandes[11]	2008	9.2 km
Mallo, et al.[5]	2007	11.1 km
Weston, et al.[12]	2006	11.62 km
Button & Peterson[13]	2005	10.43 km
Castagna & D'Ottavio[14]	2001	11.58 km
D'Ottavio & Castagna[15]	2001	11.38 km
Krustrup & Bangsbo[16]	2001	10.1 km

TABLE 3.3 Percentage of total match time of soccer referees

Authors	Year	Distance covered (km)	Standing (%)	Walking (%)	Jogging (%)	Running (%)	Sprinting (%)	Back and sideways (%)
Krustrup, et al.[3]	2009	10.270 ± 0.90	21.9 ± 4.7	40.2 ± 5.1	15.8 ± 2.9	9.3 ± 1.5 4.8 ± 1.5 2.1 ± 0.9	0.4 ± 0.2	5.3 ± 2.4 0.2 ± 0.2
Mallo, et al.[22]	2009	10.218 ± 0.64	37.1 ± 3.5	26.0 ± 1.8	20.2 ± 2.1	8.9 ± 1.2	7.7 ± 1.5	–
Mascarenhas, et al.[6]	2009	10.32 ± 4.86	Standing + Walking 65 ± 5.9		21 ± 2.8	12 ± 3.4	2 ± 1.3	–
Da Silva, Fernandes & Fernandes[11]	2008	9.156 ± 0.07	–					
Mallo, et al.[5]	2007	11.059 ± 0.94	27.4 ± 4.5	30.3 ± 2.1	25.5 ± 5.4	12.2 ± 2.3	4.6 ± 1.4	–

BOX 3.1 PHYSICAL TRAINING AND TESTING BY FIFA

The International Football Association (FIFA) has reacted to the high physical demands imposed on their referees by introducing a fitness test especially adapted to match activities. To give an example, the FIFA fitness test for referees and assistant referees consists of two tests:

1. Average running speed during repeated fast runs over a specific match distance → 6 × 40 metre sprint, with max 1.5 minutes recovery after each sprint

2. Capacity to perform repeated high-intensity runs → 20 × 150 metre sprint + 50 metre walking

Evaluation is based on reference times with different requirements for the international and national level as well as for male and female referees.[30]

Physiological responses

The preceding sections focused on the demands that are placed on referees during a competitive match. However, it is important to examine how referees actually react to these demands from a bodily standpoint. These so-called physiological responses are a good indicator of the physical fitness of a referee and can be used for individualised training and testing.

The easiest method of assessment is measuring heart rate during physical stress. Referees have shown mean values of 85–95 per cent of their maximal heart rates during competitive matches (see Castagna, Abt and D'Ottavio[2] for an overview). These relatively high heart rates show the high demands that are put on referees, which are comparable to players (85 per cent).[23] Another method is the aerobic involvement, which is measured by estimating match oxygen uptake (VO_2). Referees have been shown to attain about 70 per cent of VO_{2max}. Variations exist due to differences in capturing heart rate or oxygen uptake, such as during an actual game versus on a treadmill in the laboratory or due to different skill levels and countries. Studies conducted on a treadmill in the laboratory revealed overestimations of the actual match VO_2. Therefore, assessments during match play using a portable gas analyser should be prioritised.

In order to measure the extent to which anaerobic glycogenolysis is activated, blood lactate measurements are conducted. Blood lactate concentrations of up to 14 mmol/L have been reported for elite referees.[16] However, high variability between individuals as well as dependencies on game intensities suggest that this might not be the best indicator for referee fitness. An additional method to capture physical fitness is related to the hydration status of referees. As shown by the heart rates during competitive matches, high physical demands are put on referees that can result in significant body mass fluid losses. These can be tolerated by well-trained individuals; therefore this method might be another good indicator of physical fitness. Fluid loss is additionally influenced by environmental conditions such as heat or humidity, showing its relevance for certain leagues and competitions. Limited research has addressed this issue for referees, with only one study revealing a fluid evaporation-induced bodyweight loss of two per cent in Brazilian elite soccer referees.[24] These losses are known to negatively influence exercise as well as cognitive performance.[25] Considering World Cups and League Games in countries such as Qatar or Brazil, fluid loss should be a topic of interest for training programmes of referees.

Physical capacities

Besides the above-mentioned bodily demands placed on referees and their reactions to these demands, assessments of body compositions can provide insights into the health status and preconditions for their task. It must be considered that the career pathway of referees takes several years (often also due to previous participation as players), so that they are on average 10–15 years older than the players they are refereeing.[26] Given that referees face similar demands to those of players during games, they are required to attain excellent age-related fitness. Therefore, individualised fitness programmes are even more important to ensure that referees can keep up with play at all times and throughout the whole game. An indicator for body composition and relative body fat is the body mass index (BMI), which is based on an individual's weight and height. The BMI of referees has been measured with mean values of 24.2 kg/m^2 in elite referees participating in the Euro 2000 Championship finals. BMI values of 18.5–24.9 kg/m^2 are considered normal.[27] Physiological capacities referring to maximal oxygen uptake have rarely been examined. Summing up the few studies of this measure, however, reveals that referees show low to moderate VO$_{2max}$ values (mean of 40–50 mL/kg/min) compared with players (for an overview, see Castagna, Abt and D'Ottavio).[2] During competitive matches referees are involved in a number of sprinting activities, showing the importance of anaerobic capacities. These have been examined measuring 50 metre and 200 metre sprinting or vertical jump performance. However, strength performance in general has not been assessed, but is suggested as an additional factor for anaerobic capacities.[2]

Link between physical demands and decision making

The preceding sections have shown that interactors, especially soccer referees, face high physical strains in order to keep up with play. However, even the fittest referee still needs to show fair and accurate judgements. Therefore, the link between physical aspects and decision-making aspects of the task is crucial for refereeing performance. Although this link seems obvious, research in this field is scarce. A precondition for accurate judgements is optimal positioning in order to achieve the best available viewing perspectives (for detailed information see also Chapter 4). Due to the above-described physical demands during a competitive match, one might assume that referees experience fatigue towards the end of a game, resulting in greater distances from play.

One method of analysis is to determine the referee's distance from play and relate it to his/her judgement accuracy. De Oliveira, Orbetelli and De Barros Neto[28] reported no significant associations between the mean distance of Brazilian referees from foul play and their decision-making accuracy. On the contrary, the highest percentage of correct calls was shown at 20–25 metres from the play (however, see Box 3.2 for different results).

BOX 3.2 STUDY ON POSITIONING AND DECISION MAKING

The soccer referees' decision in relation to position was also tested during the elite senior FIFA Confederations Cup 2009.[29] The results revealed that, for the central area of the field, error percentage was not uniformly distributed in relation to the distance to the incidents. The lowest error rate was achieved with distances of 11–15 metres from incidents, quite a bit higher than that shown by De Oliveira, Orbetelli and De Barros Neto.[28] Although distance to infringements did not increase between halves and 15 minute periods, the error percentage increased from 9.3 per cent to 17 per cent from the first to the second half in the central area of the field, reaching its peak towards the end of the game.

Similarly, physical fatigue might lead to a decrease in decision-making accuracy with cumulative distance covered throughout a game. Studies have revealed an increase in the distance from infringements towards the end of the game, by analysing variations between the first and second half.[3, 16] However, again there was no relation between the quality of judgements and distance covered.[28, 6]

Given that higher movement speed is assumed to change visual perception, it is speculated that referees are influenced in their decision-making accuracy while moving at greater velocities. Although assistant referees' judgements are influenced by their movement speed (see Chapter 4), no relation was found between a soccer referee's accuracy and movement speed.[6] Nevertheless, since running at high intensities leads to fatigue in a short time, it would be of interest to examine referees' accuracy directly after several sprints. Even if referees are able to keep up with play during fast game situations, they should still be able to accurately judge foul situations, despite such quickly induced physical fatigue.

As illustrated, several possibilities exist to examine the relation between physical demands and decision making. However, so far only indirect analysis methods have been used. Future studies should address this topic more specifically by testing the direct influence of physical stress on decision-making accuracy. For instance, referees could be asked to judge video clips of soccer scenarios while running on a treadmill with similar physical demands as on the field. This could also be used for training purposes, cognitively adapting to fatigue effects.

Summary and conclusion

Taken together, we have presented different assessment methods as well as aspects of physical demands in sports officiating. A distinction has been made between activities that occur during match play, physiological responses to these activities and physical capacities. Studies have shown that soccer referees in particular have to consistently work on achieving and maintaining a high status of physical fitness in order to keep up with play. However, irrespective of physical demands on the field, judgements and decisions of sports officials still need to be accurate to ensure fair game and competition outcomes. This topic will be covered in the following chapters.

Official's call

Bill Mildenhall

This chapter addresses an area that is critical in basketball officiating: physical demands. Below I pick out and comment on some of the key areas of the chapter, relating my experience in the field, the practices that are used and their evolution.

Training and activities during match play

Based on the information from studies and my personal experiences over 30 years, it is clear that basketball officiating utilises both energy systems – endurance (aerobic) and speed/power (anaerobic). As a consequence, elite referees are aware of the need to train both systems to ensure they are in good physical condition to officiate a game.

Obviously, however, there needs to be performance beyond this level, which is why physical training is so important and has to match the demands.

Elite referees in the Australian state of Victoria did some physical studies many years ago with a university using calibrated court marking, video analysis, heart rate monitoring and fluid loss measurements. I suspect that these findings are still pretty accurate, although the athleticism of the players has increased considerably. Interestingly, FIBA (the International Controlling Body of World Basketball) acknowledged this some 25 years ago and introduced a formalised fitness testing programme using the Laser Intermittent Beep Test along with sprint tests over short distances. After some ten years the sprint test was eliminated. I am not totally sure why, but I assume it was becoming more of an additional endurance test and not really testing a referee's speed and power.

The Laser Endurance Test, as required by FIBA, does not strictly use the test in the way it was designed. FIBA set arbitrary levels that male and female referees must achieve (lower levels for female referees than for males). The test in Victoria produced some findings in terms of the distance travelled by referees and broke it down into sprint, jog and walk phases. I suspect the distance may have changed, but only minimally. The breakdown of sprint/jog/walk I suspect would be very much the same. This breakdown, of course, is dependent on a number of variables such as the style of the game, the standard of the game, the scores of the game and the ability of the referees to keep up with the requirements.

At FIBA level there has never really been a concerted effort to address the current testing programme, and consequently it has been the same for 30 years. The Australian Institute of Sport uses a variation of the Laser Intermittent Beep Test for their basketball players and have done so for the past 20 years. They use an Intermittent Yo-Yo endurance test which is believed to simulate the physical running requirements (endurance) of the elite basketball player more accurately. It is strongly suspected that the Yo-Yo test would also be more appropriate for basketball referees as it simulates some rest or walk periods during the continuous running.

Physiological responses and appearances

The testing programme conducted some 20 years ago indicated very similar results to the current testing results. Elite basketball referees train themselves or are trained informally to always appear cool and calm, particularly in a crisis or pressure situation. They pride themselves on always appearing to be in control of the game and, more importantly, in control of their emotions. Body image for a basketball referee is of paramount importance. If a referee 'looks the part', he/she will go a long way to 'being the part'. A fit, well-groomed and correctly attired referee already achieves an acceptance level before even picking up the whistle.

However, experience tells you that, in the pressure cooker situation of a tight game requiring intense concentration and above average decision-making accuracy, referees' heart rates go through the roof. Interestingly, the studies done 20 years ago had a very interesting case. The fittest elite referee (as measured by the Beep Test because, in those days, referees were encouraged to reach their maximum) was refereeing a pre-season final game which was being televised nationally and had 3,000 spectators. The game was a one point ball game, with the referee having to make a decision with only two or three seconds remaining which, either way, would determine the result of the game. He was wearing a heart rate monitor which recorded a rate above his predicted maximum. The entire time he had the appearance that this situation did not faze him in any way. I suspect his level of physical fitness contributed immensely to the position he was in to make the decision, his ability to make a decision accurately, and his ability to give the impression that he was not under any additional pressure.

Physical capacities

Basketball referees are older than the players they are officiating for the same reasons as documented in the chapter. FIBA and their 213 National Basketball Federations have a statute in place that international referees can be active in FIBA competitions up to the age of 50 years; the American Professional League (NBA) does not have any age restrictions and, as a result, have had referees up to and beyond 70 years. Studies indicate that basketball referees require at least 10,000 hours of pressurised decision-making experiences before they achieve elite referee status. This requires many years of regularly officiating high quality games. Because of the above factors and the factors already mentioned, the physical conditioning and physical capabilities of a referee will be considerably less than a player, but considerably better than the non-athletic norm.

The link between physical demands and decision making

I believe that there is an unchallenged acceptance from elite basketball referees and basketball referee-coaches that the key to accurate decision making is positioning. Referees strive to achieve the optimal position to see the play, as it is critical for accurate decision making. Referees must work to obtain a position between the players who are continually moving. Logically, if a referee is not physically capable of getting into the correct position on every play, their decision making will be compromised. This is particularly critical in the later periods of a game where it appears that the referee's decisions now can directly influence the result of the game.

Basketball referees are encouraged to be continually on the move because the players they are officiating generally never stand still. Referees should aim to anticipate the play and move appropriately so they are in a position to 'see between the players'. Referees are encouraged to move quickly into position, then adjust accordingly, avoiding making decisions while moving quickly.

Overall, this chapter was very applicable to basketball and reflected my experience of the importance of the physical demands, but also the interaction with other factors like decision making.

References

[1] Reilly, T., & Gregson, W. (2006). Special populations: The referee and assistant referee. *Journal of Sports Sciences, 24*, 795–801.

[2] Castagna, C., Abt, G., & D'Ottavio, S. (2007). Physiological aspects of soccer refereeing performance and training. *Sports Medicine, 37*, 625–46.

[3] Krustrup, P., Helsen, W., Morten, B. R., Christensen, J. F., MacDonald, C., Rebelo, A. N., & Bangsbo, J. (2009). Activity profile and physical demands of football referees and assistant referees in international games. *Journal of Sports Sciences, 27*, 1167–76.

[4] Mallo, J., & Navarro, E. (2004). Analysis of the load imposed on under-19 soccer players during typical football training drills. In: Part II: Game activity and analysis. *Journal of Sports Sciences, 22*, 500–20.

[5] Mallo, J., Navarro, E., Garcia-Aranda, J. M., Gilis, B. and Helsen, W. (2007). Activity profile of top-class association football referees in relation to performance in selected physical tests. *Journal of Sports Sciences, 25*, 805–13.

[6] Mascarenhas, D., Button, C., O'Hare, D., & Dicks, M. (2009). Physical performance and decision making in association football referees: A naturalistic study. *The Open Sports Sciences Journal, 2*, 1–9.

[7] Barbero-Alvarez, J. C., Boullosa, D. A., Nakamura, F. Y., Andrín, G., & Castagna, C. (2012). Physical and physiological demands of field and assistant soccer referees during America's Cup. *Journal of Strength and Conditioning Research, 26*, 1383–8.

[8] Weston, M., Drust, B. & Gregson, W. (2011). Intensities of exercise during match-play in FA Premier League referees and players. *Journal of Sports Sciences, 29*, 527–32.

[9] Weston, M., Drust, B., Atkinson G., & Gregson, W. (2011). Variability of soccer referees' match performances. *International Journal of Sports Medicine, 32*, 190–4.

[10] Weston, M., Castagna, C., Impellizzeri, F. M., Rampinini, E., & Breivik, S. (2010). Ageing and physical match performance in English Premier League soccer referees. *Journal of Science and Medicine in Sport, 13*, 96–100.

[11] Da Silva, A. I., Fernandes, L. C., & Fernandez, R. (2008). Energy expenditure and intensity of physical activity in soccer referees during match-play. *Journal of Science and Medicine, 7*, 327–34.

[12] Weston, M., Castagna, C., Impellizzeri, F. M., Rampinini, E., & Abt, G. (2006). Analysis of between-half work rates in English Premier League soccer referees. *Journal of Science and Medicine in Sport, 9*, 256–62.

[13] Button, C., & Petersen, C. (Eds). (2005). *Quantifying the physiological demands of football refereeing using GPS tracking technology.* Dunedin, New Zealand: University of Otago.

[14] Castagna, C., & D'Ottavio, S. (2001). Effect of maximal aerobic power on match performance in elite soccer referees. *Journal of Strength and Conditioning Research, 15*, 420–5.

[15] D'Ottavio, S., & Castagna, C. (2001). Analysis of match activities in elite soccer referees during actual match play. *Journal of Strength and Conditioning Research, 15*, 167–71.

[16] Krustrup, P., & Bangsbo, J. (2001). Physiological demands of top-class soccer refereeing in relation to physical capacity: effect of intense intermittent exercise training. *Journal of Sports Sciences, 19*, 881–91.

[17] Mallo, J., Navarro, E., Garcia Aranda, J. M., & Helsen, W. (2009). Physical demands of top-class soccer assistant refereeing during high-standard matches. *International Journal of Sports Medicine, 30*, 331–6.

[18] Kay, B., & Gill, N. D. (2003). Physical demands of elite Rugby League referees: Part 1 – Time and motion analysis. *Journal of Science and Medicine in Sport, 6*, 339–42.

[19] Martin, J., Smith, N. C., Tolfrey, K., & Jones, A. M. (2001). Activity analysis of English premiership rugby football union refereeing. *Ergonomics, 44*, 1069–75.

[20] Rebelo, A. N., Ascensão, A. A., Magalháes, J. F., Bischoff, R., Bendiksen, M., & Krustrup, P. (2011). Elite futsal refereeing: activity profile and physiological demands. *Journal of Strength and Conditioning Research, 25*, 980–7.

[21] Borin, J. P., Daniel, J. F., Bonganha, V., De Moraes, A. M., Cavaglieri, C. R., Mercadante, L. A., Da Silva, M. T. N., & Montagner, P. C. (2013). The distances covered by basketball referees in a match increase throughout the competition phases, with no change in physiological demand. *Open Access Journal of Sports Medicine, 4*, 193–8.

[22] Mallo, J., Navarro, E., Garcia-Aranda, J.-M., & Helsen, W. (2009). Activity profile of top-class association football referees in relation to fitness-test performance and match standard. *Journal of Sports Sciences, 27*, 9–17.

[23] García, O. G., Boubeta, A. R., & Deus, E. R. (2012). Using heart rate to detect high-intensity efforts during professional soccer competition. *Journal of Strength and Conditioning Research, 26*, 2058–64.

[24] Da Silva, A. I., & Fernandes, R. (2003). Dehydration of football referees during a match. *British Journal of Sports Medicine, 37*, 502–6.

[25] Maughan, R. J., & Shirreffs, S. M. (2010). Dehydration and rehydration in competative sport. *Scandinavian Journal of Medicine and Science in Sports, 20,* 40–7.

[26] Helsen, W., & Bultynck, J. B. (2004). Physical and perceptual-cognitive demands of top-class refereeing in association football. *Journal of Sports Sciences, 22,* 179–89.

[27] Kenney, W. L., Wilmore, J. H., & Costill, D. L. (Eds). (2012). *Physiology of Sport and Exercise 5th Edition.* Champaign, IL: Human Kinetics.

[28] De Oliveira, M. C., Orbetelli, R., & De Barros Neto, T. L. (2011). Call accuracy and distance from the play: A study with Brazilian soccer referees. *International Journal of Exercise Science, 4,* 30–8.

[29] Mallo, J., Frutos, P. G., Juárez, D., & Navarro, E. (2012). Effect of positioning on the accuracy of decision making of association football top-class referees and assistant referees during competitive matches. *Journal of Sport Sciences, 30,* 1437–45.

[30] Fédération Internationale de Football Association (FIFA) (2010). *Regulations on the organisation of refereeing in FIFA Member Associations.* Zürich, Switzerland.

4

VISUAL PERCEPTION

Introduction

'To see or not to see, that is the question.'

Perceiving, and in most cases seeing, is at the root of any judgement and decision in refereeing in sports. Sports officials must see before they can judge and decide, whether it concerns a tackle in soccer or the landing location of the ball in tennis. Even though several other factors play an important role (e.g., physical requirements, game management, Chapters 3 and 5; see also the social cognition approach by Plessner and Haar[1]), perception plays a large part in any decision made by sports officials. As such, perception provides the foundation on which all other aspects of officiating are built. Still, relatively little is known about the perceptual basis of refereeing decisions. In this chapter we will present the research that has tested vision and perception in officiating. First we will give a brief theoretical introduction on perception, after which we will address perceptual skill in sports and in officiating. In doing this, we will point out how crucial positioning and proper perspective are for good decision making in sports officiating. Finally we will give suggestions for the training practice of referees that emphasises perception and vision. As most of the scientific research is on interactors, especially referees in soccer, this chapter will emphasise this role. This should not be taken to imply that what is presented only applies to interactors in soccer; the principles are relevant to all officials.

Theory of perception

When we use the term 'perception', we are referring to the detection of perceptual information from the environment. Information literally informs us about the environment and our actions in it. When we detect the relevant information from the environment, we can control and coordinate our actions, such as catching or throwing a ball, or we can judge and make decisions about what we perceive – for instance, whether a tackle made by a soccer player is a foul or whether the falling attacker makes a dive. For the latter example it is important to detect or pick up the relevant information that tells us whether what happened was a foul or a dive. Does the referee actually see physical contact between the two players or does he decide on the basis of the movements of the players alone?[2, 3] In short, the basis for good decisions is the detection of relevant information about the situation.

Attention is the process with which we control which information we detect and which information we leave unattended. Because we cannot detect all the information that is available around us, we have to select the information that is relevant for our actions and decisions. Generally there are two ways in which our attention is controlled. One way is to use our intentions to steer our attention (top-down using the goal-directed attentional system[4]). For example, referees in soccer or basketball who want to determine whether or not the rules are violated (e.g., whether a foul is made) will steer attention towards the developing play (e.g., a tackle situation in soccer). In comparison, sometimes our attention is drawn by salient stimuli in the environment that may be highly relevant, for instance as they indicate imminent danger (bottom-up using the stimulus-driven attentional system[4]). For example, the referee's attention may be drawn away from the tackle situation to other stimuli in the environment, such as fireworks that explode at the other end of the pitch, as a result of which he will look to that location rather than the tackle.

Paying attention to the relevant information without being distracted by irrelevant information is one of the key components of perception in general and in refereeing. Findings in perceptual learning show that novices often initially rely on less useful information.[5, 6] At this stage, novices still have to learn to pay attention to the more useful sources of information. The useful information is the information that helps us control our actions and/or make reliable judgements about the environment.[7] Less useful information sources are not reliably related to those elements in the environment one wishes to perceive, judge or act upon. Taking the example of a foul or a dive in soccer, from a certain point of view it might seem that the two players make contact while in fact they do not. In that case, the information detected is not reliably related to the actual situation, especially if the falling player exaggerates his fall, thereby adding deceptive information to the scene.[2] Part of becoming an expert in any perceptual-motor skill, be it in sports as an athlete or as a referee, is to learn to rely on the more useful rather than less useful information.

Note that perception is not a passive process. We actively steer attention to pick up the relevant and useful information sources from the environment.[8, 9] In this process, two different points of observation (e.g., far and near) may provide different information about an event or situation that is perceived and judged, such as the tackle situation in soccer. As another example, a group of researchers[10] have shown that the observation point of assistant referees relative to the offside line was an important factor in determining the correct call. In other words, where the assistant referee stands influences how he or she sees the play and what his or her offside decision is. Of course, assistant referees are often moving up and down the side lines during the game. It's relevant to know that a moving point of observation (i.e., one that changes in time) allows for the pick-up of more information than a stationary point of observation. Thus, viewing perspective and orientation relative to the evolving play are essential ingredients in perception of sports officials and, hence, in their decision making. Before we go into depth on these issues, it is important to provide insight into what is known about perceptual skill in athletes because it forms the basis for what we know about officials.

Perceptual skill in athletes

Over the last two decades research into perceptual skill in sport has shown that (a) experts in sports often have superior perceptual skills compared with novices and intermediates, and (b) perceptual training may be used to speed up the process of perceptual learning leading to improved performance.

Superior perceptual skill of experts

Perceptual skill is a fundamental component of performance in many sports.[11] The ability to pick up information quickly and correctly to coordinate one's movement or to make appropriate decisions is often essential for good performance. For instance, perceptual skill is important for aiming at a target, for perceiving where to run to intercept a ball and for 'reading' the body language of opponents to anticipate their actions. A wide range of studies have investigated perceptual skill in sports by determining differences between experts and novices.[12]

Vision has long been an interesting topic for researchers who aim to understand sports performance. To this end, studies have looked at basic visual functions in athletes, such as static and dynamic acuity, field of view and depth perception, measured using standard optometric procedures and simple laboratory tasks. When the results of all these experiments are taken together, however, they show no systematic difference between expert and novice players.[11, 13, 14] Rather than in general and basic visual tasks, the differences in perceptual skill of expert and novice players present themselves in more sport-specific perceptual tasks. In these tasks, athletes have learned to pick up the most important information for the task. A popular paradigm that has been used since the 1980s to test sport-specific perceptual skill is to show video footage or slides of game situations to players and ask them what they recognise or recall, what they predict will happen next or what decision they would make. This method shows that experts respond more accurately and faster than novices (for a meta-analysis see Mann and coworkers[15]). Experts have learned to use visual information available earlier in time, for instance, from the opponent's movements, which enables them to anticipate ball direction earlier and produce a more timely response. Essentially, experts pick up early information and use this to start their responses earlier, giving them an advantage.

Another method used to look at the sport-specific visual skills of athletes is to track what exactly experts are looking at from the presentation through the measurement of eye movements. Eye movement tracking has shown that experts focus their gaze more on relevant information when predicting the opponent's actions or the direction of a ball.[16–19] Experts use fewer fixations of longer duration (i.e., they look at fewer cues but spend longer looking at them), which allows them to pick up the relevant information more efficiently and earlier from the evolving situation than novices. In comparison, when novices search for information to guide their actions, their eye movements are more erratic (more fixations of shorter duration).[15] These erratic fixations by novices seem to be consistent with the effects of anxiety on performance (see Chapter 7).

A limitation of using video or pictures to understand visual processing in sports is that they are very different from that which athletes are faced with in the reality of sports:[20] the stimulus presentation is two-dimensional, the viewpoint is fixed (and not always similar to that of a player), participants often use artificial responses such as pressing a button which is very different from actually performing an action like a kick, and often there is no relationship (coupling) between the video or picture and the actual action as seen on the field. To allow for a more realistic coupling between perception and action, researchers have used virtual reality programmes[21] and field experiments.[22–24] Findings show that expertise effects are even more clear when the stimulus presentation better resembles the real-world task.[25, 15, 26] It can be concluded that expert athletes have learned to attend to, pick up and use the information relevant for their sport tasks, whether it is returning or catching a ball, passing to a team mate, aiming the ball (or dart, arrow, puck or shuttle) at a target, or recognising patterns of play in complex dynamic team sports situations. As a result of these perceptual skills, expert athletes are able to respond faster and more accurately than novices. Note that in almost all cases experts have developed their perceptual skills automatically, merely through amassing experience and as part of their expertise in their particular sport, whether it is soccer or tennis (where much of the research has been conducted) or another sport. An important question is whether deliberate efforts and specific perceptual training can enhance and speed up the development of perceptual expertise.

Perceptual training for athletes

Several studies have investigated perceptual skill training programmes designed to improve or speed up the process of attaining (perceptual) expertise. It is widely accepted that perceptual skill is the result of task-specific practice rather than the physical or optometric characteristics of the visual system (see above).[27, 12, 28] The idea here is that sports experts develop perceptual skills after spending years watching, processing and responding to the information from their sport. They don't develop better general peripheral vision and they aren't born with better depth perception, for example. They take in information the same way mechanically, but they are better at choosing what to pick up and when. Because of this, sport-specific training programmes that more closely resemble reality are argued to be more effective, as skills trained in this way are more likely to transfer to real sport situations.[29] The majority of studies have employed video-based training with varying degrees of instruction and feedback.

The typical approach to training perceptual skill is to show video footage of an opponent's action from the player's perspective, possibly instruct participants to focus attention on certain information, let them assess the situation or choose a response and then give feedback on the response. Such training methods have been shown to improve anticipation skills in tennis,[30, 31] soccer,[32] volleyball[33] and badminton.[34] Furthermore, recent findings indicate that it is possible to increase psychological fidelity of video presentations of sport situations (i.e., so that they are experienced as more realistic) by showing the video at higher speeds (e.g., 1.5× the original speed).[35] Elite athletes trained with higher speed video improved earlier and maintained these improvements longer after the end of the programme. Thus, video-based training methods are practical and hold promise. Additionally, field-based approaches have been used successfully to train perception in more realistic settings.[36-40] In these studies, vision was manipulated during training either by using screens (Figure 4.1) or special glasses (Figure 4.2), or with specific instructions related to gaze behaviour and attentional focus. In both cases the results are promising, with relatively large improvements in performance (e.g., 10% increases in basketball shooting percentages).

Together the research findings from the video-based as well as the field-based work make clear that it is possible to both enhance and speed up the process of acquiring perceptual skill in sports. As the main task for referees lies in perception,

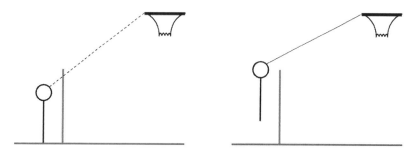

FIGURE 4.1 Graphical representation of screen training to improve basketball jump shooting.[37] In the left panel the shooter lands behind the screen for her jump shot. The screen then blocks her view to the basket. In the right panel the shooter jumps up and is able to look over the screen from about half a second before to the moment of ball release, providing just enough information for accurate shooting.[36]

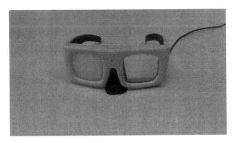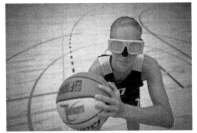

FIGURE 4.2 Plato® liquid crystal goggles that can be made transparent or opaque within milliseconds and can be used for research or training (StudioVU/ Peter Valckx©).

perceptual skill and its development in the area of officiating is of special interest here. If specific perceptual training would make it possible for referees to reach perceptual expertise earlier in their careers than is currently the case, this would be a valuable addition to their training and education.

Perceptual skill in officiating

Although decision making informed by visual perception is only one of many components of sports performance, for sports officials it is their core business. As an example, during the Euro 2000 soccer tournament, the refereeing teams on average made 137 observable decisions per match, with about 44 made by the head referee alone.[41] These decisions often have a direct impact on the outcome of the competition. Officials sometimes have to interpret players' actions based on their intentions, which requires advanced contextual judgement and emotional intelligence (see also Chapter 6 on game management). They have to evaluate fast-paced sometimes intentionally deceptive actions on the basis of very little information. When an action is perceived, it needs to be classified as legal or illegal, stored in memory or compared with other actions from memory before a decision can be made. This is why the skill of picking up key information as well as recognising typical tactics and practices is of great importance for sports officials

Expertise in refereeing

In contrast to the large number of studies on differences between expert and novice athletes, there are only a few studies on expertise differences in refereeing.[42, 43] Still, these studies have shown that more experienced referees show better decision making than less experienced referees or novices. Interestingly, in one study it was found that expert soccer referees were superior in accommodation, peripheral vision, eye movements and the speed of shape recognition than less experienced referees and a student control group.[44] A second study yielded similar results in comparing elite referees who were successful and unsuccessful on a video-based pre-test,[45] with better visual skills for the successful group than for the unsuccessful group. These results are somewhat in contrast to the results with elite or experienced athletes who were not found to have better basic visual skills than intermediates or novices. Possibly this may be explained by the fact that, rather than taking part in the action and having to control their own perceptual-motor performance (as their primary task), referees have to provide perceptual-cognitive judgements that might benefit from enhanced basic visual skills. Obviously more research is needed to gain more insight into this issue. Still, Plessner and Shallies[46] have found that experienced gymnastics judges had better judgements and were less distracted by a secondary task than laypersons. Recently, Hancock and Ste-Marie[47] have shown that higher level ice hockey referees are better at decision making than lower level referees, even though there were no differences in gaze behaviours. These results suggest that higher level referees are better at processing the relevant information for their decision making. Apparently, experienced referees have also learned to pick up the more relevant and useful information more efficiently, leading to better judgements and decisions.

Influence of positioning on perception and decision making

As indicated by MacMahon and Plessner,[48] one of the challenges for sports officials is that, in many cases, they have to decide on the basis of incomplete information or less useful information sources.[49] In some sports the position of the referees or judges is fixed. This may have an unwanted effect on decision making. Plessner and Shallies, for instance, found that, in judging gymnasts holding a cross on rings, a viewpoint that departed from a frontal view led to more errors in judging whether the arms of the athletes deviated from horizontal.[46] Thus, being in an optimal position or being able to move appropriately relative to the relevant scene (e.g., the evolving play) is essential in obtaining as much relevant information as possible. In several sports this optimal positioning is specifically organised by positioning officials in those positions providing the best perspective to execute their task. Examples are home plate umpires in baseball (behind the batter), replay officials in American Football (in the press box above the field), line umpires in tennis (looking down the line in question), and chair umpires in tennis and volleyball (high position above the court). Even in these cases, the human perceptual system is sometimes not sufficiently accurate for impeccable performance, which has led to the introduction of the Hawk Eye system in tennis and video replay possibilities in several other sports such as rugby and field hockey (see Chapter 8 for a discussion of technology in officiating).

In sports such as basketball and soccer, referees rarely judge game situations from an entirely stationary position. Due to the complex dynamic nature of, for instance, a soccer match, referees walk and run about the field to continuously occupy a proper vantage point from where the evolving play can be adequately perceived. As an aside, one consequence of this free-moving role is that the amount of physical work done by soccer referees during a match appears to be comparable to that of soccer players (see Chapter 3).[50–52] This explains the emphasis in training and selection of referees on their physical fitness and conditioning. Self-movement of referees also provides crucial information for their perceptual judgements. Changes in viewing perspective – whether evoked by locomotion, eye/head movements or both – will also affect the decisions of referees. Referees have to obtain sufficient information about the evolving play to make their judgements by moving about the field and scanning the environment with eye and head movements. Thus, moving about the field and scanning the environment are essential ingredients of successful refereeing as they allow referees to pick up both specific and contextual information that is necessary for the correct evaluation of a particular game situation.

There is, however, limited research on positioning of referees relative to evolving play. Little is known about how well referees manage to position themselves for accurate decision making. For an actual referee on the field, one would predict that there is an optimal distance to the situation in order to have a sufficient view of the evolving play (and possibly the intentions of players going for the ball or the opponent's legs) and sufficient detail to judge the specifics of the situation (e.g., whether or not there is actual contact between players in the tackle). Only two studies have recently addressed this issue, yielding ambiguous results. Whereas one study[53] did not find a relationship between distance to the scene and accuracy of decision making in soccer, a second study did.[54] In the latter study, accuracy in decision making was related to the distance of the referee from the evolving play, with distances of 11–15 metres leading to best performance (see also Box 3.1 in Chapter 3). Obviously, more research is needed to gain insight into the relationship between the distance of the (free-moving) referee from the action and the accuracy of decision making.

One type of official that has received more research attention than others over the past decades is the assistant referee in soccer. This attention has centred around the task of judging offside. It has been shown that the positioning of assistant referees relative to the offside line has important consequences for offside decisions.[10, 55–58] Without going into extensive details, roughly speaking a player is offside when s/he is positioned between the last two opponents (in most cases the second to last defender and the goalkeeper) at the moment that the ball is passed in his or her direction. Whether visual information about relative positions of the relevant players (i.e., the passer, the receiving attacker and the second to last defender) reliably informs about their actual positions depends on the position of the assistant referee at the side line and his accompanying perspective on the scene. Not being in line with the second to last defender may lead to errors in judging offside (see Box 4.1).[10, 55] Furthermore, it has been shown that, in actual top level soccer matches varying from First League matches in various European countries[55, 58] to World Cup matches,[56] assistant referees are frequently not on the offside line when making offside judgements. In fact they are only on the offside line in 13–24 per cent of the offside decisions. Otherwise, they lead and trail the offside line in 10–62 per cent and 22–55 per cent of cases, respectively. In short, not being in line with the second to last defender is part of the reality of judging offside, and it seems that at least part of the errors in judging offside are related to this mispositioning of the assistant referee and the accompanying viewing perspective.[10, 55]

BOX 4.1 THE OPTICAL ERROR HYPOTHESIS

If an assistant referee is not positioned perfectly on the offside line – that is, if he's not in line with the second last defender – he will look at the offside line and the relevant players at an angle. This gives the referee a point of view that may erroneously inform him about actual player positions. This is demonstrated in Figure 4.3. The left picture shows what a referee might see if he is positioned on the offside line. He sees the passer (white) and the second last defender (red), the latter of which is obscuring the attacker who will receive the pass. This attacker is clearly not offside. If, however, the assistant referee leads the offside line by about one metre or so, he will see the situations entirely differently, as is shown in the right picture. The receiving attacker now seems to be offside, especially if one considers the fast moving pace of the game and the split second decision the assistant referee has to make.

In short, as a result of the incorrect positioning and accompanying point of view, the assistant referee may perceive the wrong relative positions of the players on several occasions which can lead to an incorrect decision. It has been shown in several studies that the observation point of assistant referees relative to the offside line, and the corresponding viewing angle, is an important determining factor in incorrect decisions in judging offside.[10, 58] This is now called the optical error hypothesis.

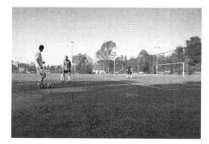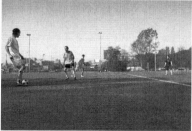

FIGURE 4.3   Same situation from two different points of view, on the offside line (left) and about a meter leading the offside line (right) (StudioVU/Yvonne Compier).

This work makes clear that, in many cases, it is difficult to obtain an optimal position, especially as the official has to make a decision about evolving play on the basis of limited information from a suboptimal perspective and often in a split second.[10, 58, 59] As mentioned in the beginning of this chapter, what the referee sees from his or her perspective provides a decisive basis for many, if not all, decisions irrespective of possible additional factors that play a role. The challenge is to learn to detect and use the relevant, yet limited, information as well as possible. Specific training may help in achieving that goal.

Perceptual training for referees

Even though perceptual skill is at the basis of the main tasks of many officials in sports, specific training of perceptual skill has received little attention, both in practice and in research. In practice there is a large emphasis on physical fitness training and testing, while perceptual skill training is largely ignored. Perceptual experience of many officials is gained purely by the experience gained in refereeing actual matches. As an aside, recent studies have shown that gaining experience as a player also helps in gaining expertise as a referee,[60] because having motor experience as a player actually helps in picking up relevant information from, for instance, the movements of players (see also research on the contribution of motor experience to perceptual skill, i.e., action-specific perception[3, 61, 62] and the discussion in Chapter 2 on the development of officials). For instance, Renden et al.[3] found that former experience as a player helped in discriminating fouls from dives in soccer tackle situations.

Several recent studies make clear that specific perceptual training using video clips is promising in improving the quality of decision making of referees. Catteeuw et al.[63] have shown that both training with video and computer animations of potential offside situations helped in improving offside judgements from pre- to post-test. In two experiments, Schweizer et al.[64] demonstrated that video training in which soccer referees watched videos, made decisions and received feedback on the correctness of their decisions improved their decision making from pre- to post test. These findings show the potential of specific perceptual training to improve referees' perception and decision making, especially as modern technologies make it easier to make video clips for training available online on computers, smart phones or tablets. What remains to be seen is to what degree the positive results from the studies transfer to the actual playing field, although a promising first step was made by Put et al.[65]

Thus, on the basis of the research findings, it seems possible to improve and enhance perception and, thus, decision making in referees and officials. We argue that, next to the traditional emphasis on physical conditioning in training of referees, one should also explicitly practice perception and decision making, which is at the core of their main task. In this regard we advise officials to focus on perceptual training, preferably from the proper perspective (i.e., match-specific). Note that training is an issue that is also addressed in Chapter 8 (Technology) and Chapter 9 (Selection, training and evaluation of performance).

Summary and conclusion

Perception, and often vision, is the basis of all officiating judgements, even if several other factors such as the crowd and game management issues play a role. So far, perceptual skill in officiating is most often acquired through experience in officiating games. Perceptual training studies in sport in general show that it is possible to speed up perceptual learning processes. The structural introduction of practice of perception and decision making into training of referees is therefore advised.

References

[1] Plessner, H., & Haar, T. (2006). Sports performance judgments from a social cognitive perspective. *Psychology of Sport and Exercise, 7,* 555–75.

[2] Morris, P. H., & Lewis, D. (2010). Tackling diving: the perception of deceptive intentions in association football (soccer). *Journal of Nonverbal Behavior, 34,* 1–13.

[3] Renden, P. G., Kerstens, S., Oudejans, R. R. D., & Cañal-Bruland, R. (2014). Foul or dive? Motor contributions to judging ambiguous foul situations in football. *European Journal of Sport Science, 14,* S221–7.

[4] Corbetta, M., & Shulman, G. L. (2002). Control of goal-directed and stimulus-driven attention in the brain. *Nature Reviews Neuroscience, 3,* 201–15.

[5] Jacobs, D. M., Runeson, S., & Michaels, C. F. (2001). Learning to visually perceive the relative mass of colliding balls in globally and locally constrained task ecologies. *Journal of Experimental Psychology: Human Perception and Performance, 27,* 1019–38.

[6] Jacobs, D. M., & Michaels, C. F. (2002). On the apparent paradox of learning and realism. *Ecological Psychology, 14,* 127–39.

[7] Beek, P. J., Jacobs, D. M., Daffertshofer, A., & Huys, R. (2003). Expert performance in sport: Views from the joint perspectives of ecological psychology and dynamical systems theory. In J. Starkes & A. Ericsson (Eds). *Expert performance in sport* (pp. 321–44). Champaign, IL: Human Kinetics.

[8] Gibson, J. J. (1986). *The ecological approach to visual perception* (first published 1979). Hillsdale, NJ: Lawrence Erlbaum Associates, Inc.

[9] Michaels, C. F., & Carello, C. (1981). *Direct perception.* Englewood Cliffs, NJ: Prentice-Hall.

[10] Oudejans, R. R. D., Verheijen, R., Bakker, F. C., Gerrits, J. C., Streinbrückner, M., & Beek, P. J. (2000). Errors in judging "offside" in football. *Nature, 404,* 33.

[11] Williams, A. M., Davids, K., & Williams, J. G. (Eds). (1999). *Visual perception and action in sport.* London: E. & F. N. Spon.

[12] Starkes, J. L., & Ericsson, K. A. (Eds). (2003). *Expert performance in sports: Advances in research on sport expertise.* Champaign, IL: Human Kinetics.

[13] Hazel, C. A. (1995). The efficacy of sports vision practice and its role in clinical optometry. *Clinical and Experimental Optometry, 78,* 98–105.

[14] Wood, J. M., & Abernethy, B. (1997). An assessment of the efficacy of sports vision training programs. *Optometry and Vision Science, 74,* 646–59.

[15] Mann, D. T., Williams, A. M., Ward, P., & Janelle, C. M. (2007). Perceptual-cognitive expertise in sport: A meta-analysis. *Journal of Sport and Exercise Psychology, 29,* 457–78.

[16] Ripoll, H., Kerlirzin, Y., Stein, J. F., & Reine, B. (1995). Analysis of information processing, decision making, and visual strategies in complex problem solving sport situations. *Human Movement Science, 14,* 325–49.

[17] Williams, A. M., Davids, K., Burwitz, L., & Williams, J. G. (1994). Visual search strategies in experienced and inexperienced soccer players. *Research Quarterly for Exercise and Sport, 65,* 127–35.

[18] Singer, R. N., Cauraugh, J. H., Chen, D., Steinberg, G. M., & Frehlich, S. G. (1996). Visual search, anticipation, and reactive comparisons between highly-skilled and beginning tennis players. *Journal of Applied Sport Psychology, 8,* 9–26.

[19] Savelsbergh, G. J., Williams, A. M., Kamp, J. V. D., & Ward, P. (2002). Visual search, anticipation and expertise in soccer goalkeepers. *Journal of Sports Sciences, 20,* 279–87.

[20] Abernethy, B., Burgess-Limerick, R., & Parks, S. (1994). Contrasting approaches to the study of motor expertise. *Quest, 46,* 186–98.

[21] Bideau, B., Kulpa, R., Vignais, N., Sébastien Brault, B., Multon, F., & Craig, C. (2010). Using virtual reality to analyze sports performance. *IEEE Computer Graphics and Applications*, *30*, 64–71.

[22] Abernethy, B., Gill, D. P., Parks, S. L., & Packer, S. T. (2001). Expertise and the perception of kinematic and situational probability information. *Perception*, *30*, 233–52.

[23] Oudejans, R. R., Michaels, C. F., & Bakker, F. C. (1997). The effects of baseball experience on movement initiation in catching fly balls. *Journal of Sports Sciences*, *15*, 587–95.

[24] Dicks, M., Button, C., & Davids, K. (2010). Examination of gaze behaviors under in situ and video simulation task constraints reveals differences in information pickup for perception and action. *Attention, Perception, and Psychophysics*, *72*, 706–20.

[25] Dicks, M., Davids, K., & Button, C. (2009). Representative design for the study of perception and action in sport. *International Journal of Sport Psychology*, *40*, 506–24.

[26] Pinder, R. A., Davids, K., Renshaw, I., & Araújo, D. (2011). Manipulating informational constraints shapes movement reorganization in interceptive actions. *Attention, Perception & Psychophysics*, *73*, 1242–54.

[27] Abernethy, B. (1988). The effects of age and expertise upon perceptual skill development in a racquet sport. *Research Quarterly for Exercise and Sport*, *59*, 210–21.

[28] Ward, P., & Williams, A. M. (2003). Perceptual and cognitive skill development in soccer: the multidimensional nature of expert performance. *Journal of Sport and Exercise Psychology*, *25*, 93–111.

[29] Williams, A. M., & Grant, A. (1999). Training perceptual skill in sport. *International Journal of Sport Psychology*, *30*, 194–220.

[30] Farrow, D., & Abernethy, B. (2002). Can anticipatory skills be learned through implicit video based perceptual training? *Journal of Sports Sciences*, *20*, 471–85.

[31] Williams, A. M., Ward, P., Knowles, J. M., & Smeeton, N. J. (2002). Anticipation skill in a real-world task: measurement, training, and transfer in tennis. *Journal of Experimental Psychology: Applied*, *8*, 259–70.

[32] Williams, A. M., & Burwitz, L. (1993). Advance cue utilization in soccer. In T. Reilly, J. Clarys, & A. Stibe (Eds), *Science and football II* (pp. 239–44). London: E. & F. N. Spon.

[33] Adolphe R. M., Vickers J. N., La Plante G. (1997). The effects of training visual attention on gaze behavior and accuracy. *International Journal of Sports Vision*, *4*, 28–33.

[34] Hagemann, N., Strauss, B., & Cañal-Bruland, R. (2006). Training perceptual skill by orienting visual attention. *Journal of Sport and Exercise Psychology*, *28*, 143–58.

[35] Lorains, M., Ball, K., & MacMahon, C. (2013). Expertise differences in a video decision-making task: Speed influences on performance. *Psychology of Sport and Exercise*, *14*, 293–7.

[36] Oudejans, R.R.D. (2012). Effects of visual control training on the shooting performance of elite female basketball players. *International Journal of Sports Science and Coaching*, *7*, 469–80.

[37] Oudejans, R. R. D., Koedijker, J. M., Bleijendaal, I., & Bakker, F. C. (2005). The education of attention in aiming at a far target: Training visual control in basketball jump shooting. *International Journal of Sport and Exercise Psychology*, *3*, 197–221.

[38] Vine, S. J., & Wilson, M. R. (2011). The influence of quiet eye training and pressure on attention and visuo-motor control. *Acta Psychologica*, *136*, 340–6.

[39] Vine, S. J., Moore, L. J., & Wilson, M. R. (2014). Quiet eye training: The acquisition, refinement and resilient performance of targeting skills. *European Journal of Sport Science*, *14*(Suppl 1), S235–42.

[40] Harle, S. K., & Vickers, J. N. (2001). Training quiet eye improves accuracy in the basketball free throw. *Sport Psychologist, 15,* 289–305.

[41] Helsen, W., & Bultynck, J. B. (2004). Physical and perceptual-cognitive demands of top-class refereeing in association football. *Journal of Sports Sciences, 22,* 179–89.

[42] Bard, C., Fleury, M., Carrière, L., & Hallé, M. (1980). Analysis of gymnastics judges' visual search. *Research Quarterly for Exercise and Sport, 51,* 267–73.

[43] Ste-Marie, D. M. (2000). Expertise in women's gymnastics judging: An observational approach. *Perceptual and Motor Skills, 90,* 543–6.

[44] Ghasemi, A., Momeni, M., Rezaee, M., & Gholami, A. (2009). The difference in visual skills between expert versus novice soccer referees. *Journal of Human Kinetics, 22,* 15–20.

[45] Ghasemi, A., Momeni, M., Jafarzadehpur, E., Rezaee, M., & Taheri, H. (2011). Visual skills involved in decision making by expert referees. *Perceptual and Motor Skills, 112,* 161–71.

[46] Plessner, H., & Schallies, E. (2005). Judging the cross on rings: a matter of achieving shape constancy. *Applied Cognitive Psychology, 19,* 1145–56.

[47] Hancock, D.J., & Ste-Marie, D.M. (2013) Gaze behaviors and decision making accuracy of higher- and lower-level ice hockey referees. *Psychology of Sport and Exercise, 14,* 66–71.

[48] *MacMahon, C., & Plessner, H. (2013). The sport official in research and practice.* In D. Farrow, J. Baker & C. MacMahon (Eds.), *Developing Sport Expertise, 2nd Edition* (pp. 71–95). London: Routledge.

[49] Barte, J., & Oudejans, R. R. D. (2012). The effects of additional lines on a football field on assistant referees' positioning and offside judgments. *International Journal of Sports Science and Coaching, 7,* 481–92.

[50] Krustrup, P., Helsen, W., Randers, M. B., Christensen, J. F., MacDonald, C., Rebelo, A. N., & Bangsbo, J. (2009). Activity profile and physical demands of football referees and assistant referees in international games. *Journal of Sports Sciences, 27,* 1167–76.

[51] Mallo, J., Navarro, E., Garcia-Aranda, J. M., Gilis, B., & Helsen, W. (2007). Activity profile of top-class association football referees in relation to performance in selected physical tests. *Journal of Sports Sciences, 25,* 805–13.

[52] Mallo, J., Navarro, E., Aranda, J. M. G., & Helsen, W. F. (2009). Activity profile of top-class association football referees in relation to fitness-test performance and match standard. *Journal of Sports Sciences, 27,* 9–17.

[53] Oliveira, M. C., Orbetelli, R., & Barros, T. L. N. (2011). Call accuracy and distance from the play: A study with Brazilian soccer referees. *International Journal of Exercise Science, 4,* 30–8.

[54] Mallo, J., Frutosa, P.G., Juáreza, D., & Navarroa, E. (2012). Effect of positioning on the accuracy of decision making of association football top-class referees and assistant referees during competitive matches. *Journal of Sports Sciences, 30,* 1437–45.

[55] Catteeuw, P., Gilis, B., Wagemans, J., & Helsen, W. (2010). Offside decision making of assistant referees in the English Premier League: Impact of physical and perceptual-cognitive factors on match performance. *Journal of Sports Sciences, 28,* 471–81.

[56] Catteeuw, P., Gilis, B., Garcia-Aranda, J. M., Tresaco, F., Wagemans, J., & Helsen, W. (2010). Offside decision making in the 2002 and 2006 FIFA World Cups. *Journal of Sports Sciences, 28,* 1027–32.

[57] Gilis, B., Helsen, W., Catteeuw, P., Van Roie, E., & Wagemans, J. (2009). Interpretation and application of the offside law by expert assistant referees: Perception

of spatial positions in complex dynamic events on and off the field. *Journal of Sports Sciences, 27*, 551–63.

[58] Oudejans, R. R. D., Bakker, F. C., Verheijen, R., Steinbrückner, M., Gerrits, J. C., & Beek, P. J. (2005). How position and motion of expert assistant referees in soccer relate to the quality of their offside judgements during actual match play. *International Journal of Sport Psychology, 36*, 3–21.

[59] Plessner, H., Schweizer, G., Brand, R., & O'Hare, D. (2009). A multiple-cue learning approach as the basis for understanding and improving soccer referees' decision making. In M. Raab, J. Johnson, & H. Heekeren (Eds). *Progress in brain research: Mind and motion: The bidirectional link between thought and action* (pp. 151–8). Amsterdam: Elsevier Press.

[60] MacMahon, C., Starkes, J. L., & Deakin, J. (2009). Differences in processing of game information in basketball players, coaches and referees. *International Journal of Sport Psychology, 40*, 403–23.

[61] Cañal-Bruland, R., Kreinbucher, C., & Oudejans, R. R. D. (2012). Motor experience influences strike and ball judgments in baseball. *International Journal of Sport Psychology, 43*, 137–52.

[62] Pizzera, A., & Raab, M. (2012). Perceptual judgments of sports officials are influenced by their motor and visual experience. *Journal of Applied Sport Psychology, 24*, 59–72.

[63] Catteeuw, P., Gilis, B., Wagemans, J., & Helsen, W. (2010). Perceptual-cognitive skills in offside decision making: expertise and training effects. *Journal of Sport and Exercise Psychology, 32*, 828–44.

[64] Schweizer, G., Plessner, H., Kahlert, D., & Brand, R. (2011). A video-based training method for improving soccer referees' intuitive decision-making skills. *Journal of Applied Sport Psychology, 23*, 429–42.

[65] Put, K., Wagemans, J., Jaspers, A., & Helsen, W. F. (2013). Web-based training improves on-field offside decision-making performance. *Psychology of Sport and Exercise, 14*, 577–85.

5

JUDGEMENT AND DECISION MAKING

Introduction

Proficient judgement and decision-making skills are surely at the heart of what makes good and excellent officiating. However, at the beginning of this chapter we would like to emphasise the fact that the judgement and decision making (JDM) tasks of officials depend heavily on the rule book for each sport. Therefore, the rules need to be considered first before officials' JDM can be evaluated. For example, it makes no sense to blame the race jury for its decision to stop the 13th race of the 2013 America's Cup when Team New Zealand was little more than one nautical mile from the finish line and winning the trophy. Even if this decision appeared overly dramatic and unfair at first, there is a rule that no race should last more than 40 minutes and this time limit had expired. Thus, the jury had no choice. Unfortunately for Team New Zealand, this rule book decision gave way to an epic comeback of the Oracle Team USA which in the end won the trophy after winning eight races in a row.

Pointing to the significance of a sport's rules also makes it clear that JDM depends heavily on officials' knowledge of these rules. Although the acquisition of rule knowledge is an important component in officials' development to become experts (see Chapter 2), in some sports (e.g., gymnastics, cricket) the rules are so complicated that even the best officials sometimes fail to recall them correctly and, thus, are not able to apply them accordingly.

In Chapter 2 we also introduced the classification of officials as reactors, monitors and interactors. It depends partly on the number of players and cues (high versus low) that needs to be monitored. Among other variations between types of officials, this means that officials' JDM processes differ in terms of complexity. When comparing the decision of whether a ball in tennis was in or out with the decision of whether a football player intentionally touched the ball with his hand in soccer, it becomes obvious that different levels of cognitions are involved. According to a general theoretical approach to judging sport performance,[1] it is useful to differentiate in this area between several subtasks of information processing: perception, categorisation, memory and information integration (see Figure 5.1). These processes lead from the actual performance (e.g., a tackle in soccer) to a decision (e.g., sending a player off the field). An erroneous decision can stem from errors at different processing stages – for example, from the misperception that a player hit his opponent's leg instead of the ball or from the false memory that the player has persistently infringed the rules of the game before this situation and is now due for a strong punishment. In order to prevent such an error, it is necessary to know *why* it occurs. Chapter 4 focused on perception as a prerequisite for proficient decision-making processes. This chapter deals mainly with the processes that come later – namely, memory and information integration.

Unfortunately, most research in the area of JDM focuses on officials' systematic errors or biases rather than on their achievements. Of course they receive public attention for (obvious) decision errors rather than for their extraordinary skills. In fact, it is a widely held assumption that officials' decisions are prone to systematic, cognitive biases of which they are at least partly unaware. It is possible that some misjudgements are also products of strategic deliberation. However, we assume that in most of the cases – at least in the moment of their decision – officials are convinced that their decision is accurate and adequate. But the focus on errors in the research is also due to a specific research tradition according to which the detection of systematic errors in human cognition can help to unveil and understand

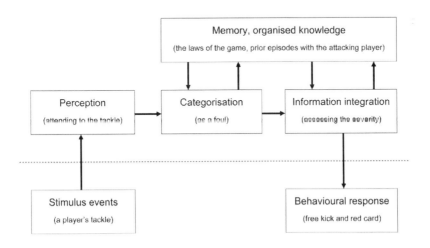

FIGURE 5.1 Information processing. Reprinted from Plessner and Haar[1] with permission from Elsevier.

the underlying processes. This would be a first step in order to improve officials' decision making. However, when talking about errors in officials' decision making, the question must arise: what is the standard of comparison? Or, is there always a correct decision in accordance with the rule book? In Chapter 6 we will learn that, at least in sport games, there is frequently an adequate decision beyond the accurate one and it is not always clear which of these two is the 'better' option. In most of the research that is reported in this chapter, officials' decisions are either compared with expert assessments (who mostly had more time to observe the situation in question) or with their own or other officials' decisions under different circumstances.

Biased decision making

There has been considerable research investigating a variety of (unwanted) factors that may affect officials' decisions, from the impact of players' shirt colour[2] to the influence of crowd noise.[3] In the following we will report some of this research, organised using the steps of information processing as proposed previously (see Figure 5.1).

Categorisation and prior knowledge

Once an action has been perceived (see Chapter 4), it needs to be encoded and given meaning (e.g., a perceived body movement is recognised as a somersault). Importantly, this information processing step relies heavily on prior knowledge (e.g., a gymnastics judge must know what a somersault looks like). The encoded movement will be stored automatically in memory and may influence future judgements, just as the activated knowledge influences current processing.

However, as in perception, there are some basic principles that influence the process of categorisation. For example, the German researchers Christian Unkelbach and Daniel Memmert found that referees in soccer games do not award as many yellow cards in the beginning of a game as should be statistically expected.[4] This can be explained by a classic model of categorisation processes. In accordance with this model, they argue that this effect arises in order to deal with the judgement situation: referees need to calibrate a judgement scale and essentially get a feel for the game. They need to make sure that they can move both up and down the scale, and so they avoid making extreme category judgements in the beginning (i.e., yellow cards). If they start with a yellow card early in a game, they would probably end up with many additional cards in order to stay consistent. For example, the World Cup match between Cameroon and Germany in 2002 resulted in a record of 14 yellow cards. In fact, the first yellow card in this game was awarded against Cameroon's midfielder Marc Vivien Foé in the eighth minute.

In many sports, officials, athletes and spectators alike hold the view that having experience as an athlete in that sport is useful – if not essential – for proficient officiating. For example, it has frequently been claimed that certain incidents on a soccer pitch can only be accurately assessed by a referee who has past playing experience. In recent years, this assumption has gained some theoretical support through the so-called embodiment perspective. It emphasises the significance of the mind's connections to the physical world. Consequently, perceptual and motor systems are considered to be highly relevant for the understanding of central cognitive processes such as judgement and decision making. For example, prior motor experiences with certain movements have been found to facilitate the recognition of these movements when performed by other people. Thus, it appears to be quite plausible to assume a positive relationship between prior specific sport experiences and officials' performance. In some sports, prior success as an athlete is even an official requirement for becoming an official on a higher level (see Chapter 9). However, the systematic investigation of officials' decision making from the viewpoint of an embodiment perspective has begun only recently. For example, Chapter 2 mentioned research in this area in gymnastics and soccer. In addition, the same researchers examined the relationship between previous motor and visual experience and officiating performance in a sample of 370 sports officials from soccer, handball, ice hockey and trampoline.[5] They found that officiating performance is related to motor, visual and officiating experience to different degrees in the analysed sports. They suggest that, depending on the sport, officials should either specialise early in officiating or gather visuo-motor experience as an athlete or spectator first, and then switch roles to become a sports official. Thus, their main finding is that gathering prior experience as an athlete is not automatically an advantage for an official in all sports.

While prior knowledge about judgement criteria in a sport and adequate categorisation systems are necessary requirements for accurate performance judgements (see above), we focus our overview on research about the use of inappropriate knowledge – that is, knowledge that has a distorting or biasing influence on judges' cognitive processes and subsequent decisions.

The colour of players' shirts has also been studied to see if it has an impact on referee perceptions and subsequent decisions. British researchers found that soccer players wearing red shirts were viewed more positively than players wearing white shirts.[6] Research has also shown that referees perceive NHL and NFL players in black shirts as more aggressive and are thus more likely to penalise them.[2] A similar finding was discovered by the German sport scientists Norbert Hagemann, Bernd Strauss and Jan Leißing[7] in Tae kwon do. In an experiment, they asked the officials to indicate how many points they would award red and blue competitors who were presented in videotaped excerpts from sparring rounds. The video clips were manipulated and edited in such a way that, for half of the referees, the colours of the competitors were reversed (e.g., player on left in red, player on right in blue versus left in blue, right in red). The results showed that the competitor wearing red protective gear was awarded on average 13 per cent more points than the competitor wearing blue protective gear. This could at least partly explain the more general finding that wearing red sports attire has a positive impact on one's outcome in a combat sport.[8]

An investigation into soccer referees showed there was no causal link between perceptions of aggressiveness and the number of penalties awarded.[9] This study revealed no changes in the number of decisions awarded against teams with an aggressive reputation, but referees were found more likely to award more severe penalties (i.e., red or yellow card) to these teams. Even though this may appear to be a 'flawed' bias in the referees' decisions, it could actually be a very functional piece of 'preventive refereeing', a referee attribute that has been deemed crucial for top flight refereeing.[10]

The encoding of information about sport performances has also been found to be influenced by categories that evolve directly from the competitive environment. For example, in gymnastics, the fact that gymnastics coaches typically place their athletes in rank order from poorest to best leads to an expectation about performance. These expectations have been found to create a bias in the evaluation of athletes in a number of sports (e.g., gymnastics, figure skating and synchronised swimming). In an experiment following this line of research, Henning Plessner investigated the thinking patterns that drive these expectations in gymnastics judging.[11] Gymnastics judges were asked to score videotaped routines of a men's team competition. The target routines appeared in either the first or the fifth position of the within-team order. Depending on how hard the judgement task was, the order had an effect: the same routine received lower scores when placed in the first position than when placed in the last position. The study also found that the categorisation of perceived value parts (i.e., the attributed difficulty to single gymnastics elements) was biased by judges' expectations.

Other sources of expectancies beyond the reputation of an athlete or a team that have been found to influence officials' judgements and decisions are, for example, stereotypes about race[12] and players' height.[13] A number of studies have even investigated gender biases in regional-level sports officials, concluding that not only are male soccer and handball players more likely to demonstrate more aggressive behaviour than females but also that male referees penalise more frequently in female soccer and handball games than in male games.[14] However, such laboratory-based studies may cloud the impact of game management (see Chapter 6) where referees rely on previous decisions to provide clarity on the boundaries between legal and illegal play.

Accordingly, a study was conducted to look at what happens in actual top-level handball games (French division one, both male and female games).[15] The analysis showed the same gender bias, though the effect was only found for more common or typically occurring decisions (nine metre throw) whereas relatively infrequent and more consequential decisions (seven metre throw) revealed no gender bias.

Although these 'biasing' influences have been treated in the literature mainly as unwelcome, it should be remembered, however, that expectancies that mirror true differences can also improve accuracy in complex judgement tasks. For example, let us go back to the study on expectancy biases in judging gymnastics described above. In most competitions, coaches indeed place their athletes in rank order from poorest at the beginning to best at the end and they perform accordingly. That means the simple judgement strategy of just lifting the score from athlete to athlete a little bit would lead to quite accurate judgements. Thus, the corresponding expectancies may help officials to adjust their judgements and decision to factual performances. However, problems arise with this strategy if athletes' performances unexpectedly deviate from their standards. Therefore, it is important for officials to recognise these cases.

Taken together, the encoding and categorisation of a perceived performance has been found to be systematically influenced by the activation of various types of prior knowledge, even when this knowledge has no performance-relevant value in judging an athlete's performance. It is clear that these influences increase in likelihood as judging situations increase in ambiguity. However, ambiguous unclear situations occur quite often in sport competitions.

While the studies reported so far demonstrate that judgements of performance are potentially biased by the activation of general memory structures like expectancies, there is also some evidence for direct memory influences on the judgement of sport performances. Such influences have been studied in an impressive series of experiments by the Canadian researcher Diane Ste-Marie and her colleagues. They investigated how the memory of prior encounters with an athlete's performance can influence actual performance judgements. In these experiments, a paradigm was developed that mirrors the warm-up/competition setting in gymnastics. In the first phase of the experiment, judges watched a series of gymnasts perform a simple element and decided whether the performance was perfect or flawed. The judges' task was the same in the second phase that followed, except that the gymnastic elements shared a relationship with the items shown in the first phase. Some of the gymnasts were shown during the second phase with the identical performance as in the first phase (e.g., both times perfect), and others were shown with the opposite performance (e.g., first perfect and then flawed). When the performance in the first and second phases differed, perceptual judgements were less accurate than when performances were the same for both phases.[16] These memory-influenced biases occurred even with a week break between the first and second phases[17] and irrespective of the cognitive task that the judges had to perform during the first phase.[18] The robustness of this effect supports the authors' assumption that perceptual judgements, such as in judging gymnastics, inevitably rely on retrieval from memory for prior episodes. Thus, the only way to avoid these biases would be to prevent judges from seeing the gymnasts perform before a competition.

Information integration

In the next step of information processing (see Figure 5.1), information about an athlete's performance that has been encoded and categorised together with information that has been retrieved from memory are integrated into a judgement. Ideally, an official considers all the relevant information for a judgement task at hand and integrates this information in the most appropriate analytical way. But humans have limits. We have a limit to how much information we can process. As well, sport situations often introduce factors such as time pressure. In fact, people frequently use short cuts to cope with complex judgement situations. For example, in the context of discussing information outside the observable performance, the official's role in the home advantage has frequently been explored. The home advantage is the idea that athletes are assumed to perform better in their home venue, in front of their home crowd. The effect of the home advantage is well established in research literature, however we are still uncertain about the factors that cause it. Many ideas have been put forward to explain its existence, which have been divided into location effects (including travel fatigue and familiarity/routines) and psychological effects (including crowd and motivation factors). Although there is little evidence to suggest the home pitch (in soccer) itself creates an advantage, it has been proposed that simply feeling that you have an advantage may be enough to give you an advantage. The referee's impact upon home advantage has been shown through work in which referees tend to award more penalties to the home team in soccer than the away team.[19] Of course, this effect could be because the home team attacks more. However, research has also looked at penalty appeals by players, and showed that the likelihood of players being awarded in a penalty appeal is 81 per cent for the home team and only 51 per cent for the away team.[20]

Another factor is the crowd. For example, British researchers investigated whether crowd noise has an influence on soccer referees' decisions concerning potential foul situations.[21] They assumed that referees have learned to use crowd noise as a decision cue because, in general, it may serve as a useful indicator for the seriousness of the foul. However, the use of this knowledge may be inappropriate and may contribute to the well-confirmed phenomenon of a home advantage in team sports, because the reaction of a crowd is usually biased against the away team. In an experiment, referees assessed various challenges videotaped from a match in the English Premier League. Half of the referees observed the video with the original crowd noise audible whereas the other half viewed the video in silence. The presence or absence of crowd noise had an effect on decisions made by the referees. Most importantly, referees who viewed challenges in the noise condition awarded significantly fewer fouls against the home team than those observing the video in silence. The authors concluded that this effect might be partly due to short-cut judgement processes in which the salient, yet potentially biased, judgement of the crowd served as a decision cue for referees. A more recent series of studies[3] presented convincing evidence for this assumption. Among other points, these studies demonstrate how biased referee decisions can contribute to the phenomenon of a home advantage in sports. Another study on the home advantage in European championship boxing found an increase in the home advantage depending on the involvement of officials:[22] the probability of a home win was 0.57 for knockouts (with little involvement), 0.66 for technical knockouts (with some involvement) and 0.74 for points decisions (with full involvement).

Again we must remember that referees are human, so it is perhaps inevitable that there will be bias. So, given that referees are required to appear fair and equitable, it is perhaps understandable (if not acceptable) that the increased pressure from home fans has an impact on them. The very same idea perhaps explains the belief that Michael Jordan (the most dominant basketball player in the NBA in the 1990s) appeared to get away with more minor infractions (e.g., travelling violations) than any other player.[23] Put another way, would you be the referee to disallow a mind-blowing reverse tomahawk dunk because Michael took an extra half step while driving to the basket? So, despite the complexity of the causes of the home advantage, it is fair to assume that the referee does influence it. Although there are pockets of excellent research in this area, we are challenged with either designing laboratory-based studies (frequently using video), which often reduce the 'real-world' idiosyncrasies that may influence referees, or developing more naturalistic studies, which can be difficult to attribute to home advantage or any other range of biases that have been shown to impact the referee. Regardless, we would welcome more research in this important area.

Some other studies show that referees are not only influenced by situational cues but by their own prior decisions. For example, in an experimental study Henning Plessner and Tilmann Betsch found a negative contingency between soccer referees' successive penalty decisions concerning the same team.[24] This means that the probability of awarding a penalty to a team decreased when they had awarded a penalty to this team in a similar situation before and increased when they had not. The opposite effect occurred with successive penalty decisions concerning first one and then the other team. Similar results have been found with basketball referees when contact situations were presented in their original game sequence, but not when they were presented as random successions of individual scenes.[25] An impressive analysis of field data from about 13,000 soccer matches presented further evidence for a tendency towards 'compensation' decisions in penalty kick decisions of referees.[26] Among other findings, this work showed that the number of two-penalty matches is larger than expected by chance and that, among these matches, there are considerably more matches in which each team is awarded one penalty than would be expected on the basis of independent penalty kick decisions. Additional analyses based on the score in the match before a penalty is awarded and on the timing of penalties suggest that awarding a penalty first to one team decreased the likelihood of another penalty for the same team and increases the corresponding likelihood for the other team. Together, these effects may be partly due to referees' goal of being fair (or consistent) in the management of a game (see Chapter 6). This can also result in so-called conformity effects.[27] Acting in highly uncertain environments, referees frequently encounter incidents which are hard to judge. In these situations, and even more when a 'team' of officials has to decide, it is desirable that they adhere to a common standard and/or conform with each other (see the example in Box 5.1).

BOX 5.1 TEAM DECISIONS

It was in the final of the German Ultimate Frisbee Indoor Nationals in 2013 when the rival teams from Heidelberg and Munich met once again in a fiercely contested game. Both teams were keeping pace with each other, trading points and putting on a show for the audience with spectacular throws and catches. In the last phase of the game the score was tied at 11:11 when Munich sent the disc across the whole field towards a player sprinting into the endzone. He went up and, despite being well defended, made an outstanding effort to catch the disc high above the ground. The audience cheered loudly because of this athletic display, however, the player did not start to celebrate after the catch. His defender immediately pointed to the side line indicating that the Munich player had landed out of bounds and therefore had not scored a goal. This is nothing extraordinary and player complaints about infractions of the opponents can be found in almost every sport. However, Ultimate Frisbee has a unique characteristic – it is the only team sport that does not use referees even at the highest national or international level. In Ultimate Frisbee, the task of the referee – with all the power and the duties to observe the rules – lies with the players themselves. The astonishing thing about this fact is that this renunciation of referees actually works in this sport. As a consequence, in the situation described above there was no mass confrontation or wild accusations to change the call of the decision maker. The two players involved – the player who caught the disc and his defender who called him out of bounds – exchanged their points of view calmly, despite the fact that this decision had a large impact on the outcome of the game. They could not agree on a decision and therefore asked for input from the surrounding players from both teams, who had a better perspective on this sweeping challenge. Taking all of the information into account, six players, team mates and opponents, stated their opinions and the Munich player accepted that he had landed on the line and therefore out of bounds. Instead of an important goal for Munich, Heidelberg was now in possession of the disc. They scored a goal in the other endzone and went on to win the National Championship 15:13.

The judgement of an athlete's performance is frequently based on the comparison with other athletes or with prior judgements of other athletes' performances. Recent research suggests that the consequences of such comparisons are tied to the specific mechanism of similarity and dissimilarity testing.[28] This means that starting the comparison process with the focus on similarities increases the likelihood of an assimilation judgement towards the standard of comparison. The focus on dissimilarities, however, is more likely to end up in a contrast effect away from a standard. These assumptions have been applied in an experiment to the judgement of gymnastics routines on the vault by experienced judges.[29] Two athletes were introduced to the judges as belonging either to the same national team (similarity focus) or to different teams (dissimilarity focus). Both gymnasts' routines had to be evaluated in a sequence. While the second routine was the same in all conditions, half of the participants first saw a better routine (high standard) while the other half first saw a worse routine (low standard). As predicted, the second gymnast's score was assimilated towards the standard when both gymnasts were introduced as belonging to the same team. The opposite effect occurred when the judges believed the gymnasts belonged to different teams. So the same gymnast was scored differently depending on general comparison processes.

Improving officials' JDM

As stated at the beginning of this chapter, the most basic requirement for officials' JDM is knowledge of the rules and laws of the sport. Hence, they are required to have a strong foundation of declarative knowledge, which is often defined as rulebook knowledge. The implementation of the rules is referred to as procedural (how to) knowledge. To learn the rules and rule application (the factual JDM), most sports provide material in the form of commentaries and accompanying videos that help the novice official to become familiar with the specific rule system beyond the mere study of the written rules. For example, a corresponding training tool has been developed on a sound theoretical basis for soccer referees' foul decisions.[30] These and similar tools are described in detail in Chapter 9. Among others, these are important because laws are typically written with the main purpose of being exact and not of being user-friendly. In addition, in some sports, learning the rules is already the greatest challenge for the future official. For example, the code of points in gymnastics is rather complex and comprises, among other things, a detailed list of hundreds of value parts that need to be recognised in a competition. Again, it seems that this kind of knowledge is not attained as an automatic consequence of mere experience in a sport – for example as an athlete – but it is acquired through specific, structured and effortful training. Apart from video material that can be helpful in order to learn both the rules and how to implement them, officials are also advised to observe and discuss athletes' performances frequently, either in training sessions or competitions.

In addition, it is important to identify key decisions, typical areas of difficulty and even sources of error. As has been discussed above, the information processing approach is helpful to identify the stage at which errors have occurred. Once again, key decisions may differ by level of play and undoubtedly for different types of decision-making systems (e.g., panel of judges versus on-field referee). This type of analysis can provide information on common practices, types of systems and their influences on decision making – for example, the use of a panel of judges responsible for providing a global mark for an athlete versus split responsibilities (e.g., technical and artistic assessments as in gymnastics).

Summary and conclusion

We started this chapter with the notion that good JDM is at the heart of what makes good and excellent officiating. However, so far, the majority of research on this issue is concerned with officials' errors – just as the public opinion. For example, some studies even provide some evidence that biased decision making by officials contributes to the home team advantage in sport. Instead of complaining about this fact, officials are well advised to take the scientific knowledge about the potential sources of erroneous decision making and develop corresponding measures in order to improve their skills. Recent research on JDM training tools opens some promising venues in this direction (see also Chapter 9). Of course, it must be kept in mind that, so far, most training tools aim at increasing officials' accuracy, which is not the only goal of their decision making, as we learn in the following chapter.

Official's call

Ralf Brand

It is a part of the official's role that they are expected to be perfect. They are accustomed to the fact that they mainly get feedback on the things that were not perfect. Therefore, I find it very polite that the authors almost apologise for speaking mainly about the biases that make officials' decisions worse. No problem, we officials can bear this; we are even particularly interested in this topic! This is even more the case if we consider the authors' argument that it would be desirable to use the knowledge about biases to make referees (even) better.

However, after reading the chapter, I have a burning interest in the question of how such biases actually affect officials' decisions. I have this question because officials on the field don't make decisions that can be affected by a bias. Rather, they decide categorically: call or no call. The decision is correct or incorrect (at best unfortunate, but certainly not a bit incorrect). Thus my question to the researchers is: if they pursue the claim that they want to make officials really better, in what percentage of an official's calls in a match (including the situations with a decision not to whistle) does a bias lead to a wrong decision? As an official I would find it much easier to accept that such research is also of practical importance if I have an idea of how many errors I could avoid in a game when I train accordingly. This is certainly not an easy task for the respective research. However, from my perspective, this is a very important one.

A second point is that officials' decisions always have two functions: first, they are a commentary on what has just happened (for example, that was good/rule-compliant or not good/not rule-compliant) and, second, and very important from an official's perspective, it's a message about how to continue – namely, "That is how we can go on" or "What you have just done is forbidden, you should not do it again (otherwise you are going to be punished/poorly rated again)". In most of the research so far, only the retrospective perspective has been considered. Shouldn't it also include the prospective perspective? To pick an example from the chapter, when it comes to the step error by Michael Jordan, even the non-decisions of the referee require some comment. Each player will accept that the marginal (step) error is not called if the monster slam dunk is successful. But none of the other (normal) players will infer that he is allowed to make the same error the next time he makes a simple lay-up. From the prospective perspective, everything depends on the sense behind the rules that is communicated in a particular context by an official. Experienced players and coaches are excellent in recognising the prospective meaning of officials' decisions and rely on officials' consistency during a game. Referees know that and use (or at least try to use) their calls/no-calls for this purpose. In my opinion, it is an important task of future research about officials' JDM to include these prospective aspects in the corresponding models of officials' behaviour.

References

[1] Plessner, H., & Haar, T. (2006). Sports performance judgments from a social cognition perspective. *Psychology of Sport and Exercise*, 7, 555–75.

[2] Frank, M. G., & Gilovich, T. (1988). The dark side of self- and social perception: Black uniforms and aggression in professional sports. *Journal of Personality and Social Psychology*, *54*, 74–85.

[3] Unkelbach, C., & Memmert, D. (2010). Crowd noise as a cue in referee decisions contributes to the home advantage. *Journal of Sport and Exercise Psychology*, *32*, 483–98.

[4] Unkelbach, C., & Memmert, D. (2008). Game-management, context-effects, and calibration: 'The case of yellow cards in soccer'. *Journal of Sport and Exercise Psychology*, *30*, 95–109.

[5] Pizzera, A., & Raab, M. (2012). Perceptual judgments of sports officials are influenced by their motor and visual experience. *Journal of Applied Sport Psychology*, *24*, 59–72.

[6] Greenlees, I., Leyland, A., Thelwell, R., & Filby, W. (2008). Soccer penalty takers' uniform color and pre-penalty kick gaze affect the impressions formed of them by opposing goalkeepers. *Journal of Sports Sciences*, *26*, 569–76.

[7] Hagemann, N., Strauss, B., & Leißing, J. (2008). When the referee sees red. *Psychological Science*, *19*, 769–71.

[8] Hill, R. A., & Barton, R. A. (2005). Red enhances human performance in contests. *Nature*, *435*, 293.

[9] Jones, M. V., Paull, G. C., & Erskine, J. (2002). The impact of a team's aggressive reputation on the decisions of association football referees. *Journal of Sports Sciences*, *20*, 991–1000.

[10] Topp, W. (1999). Managing conflict, In J. Grunska (Ed). *Successful sports officiating* (pp. 61–84), Champaign, IL: Human Kinetics.

[11] Plessner, H. (1999). Expectation biases in gymnastics judging. *Journal of Sport and Exercise Psychology*, *21*, 131–44.

[12] Stone, J., Perry, Z. W., & Darley, J. M. (1997). White men can't jump: Evidence for the perceptual confirmation of racial stereotypes following a basketball game. *Basic and Applied Social Psychology*, *19*, 291–306.

[13] Van Quaquebeke, N. & Giessner, S. R. (2010). How embodied cognitions affect judgments: Height-related attribution bias in football foul calls. *Journal of Sport and Exercise Psychology*, *32*, 3 22.

[14] Souchon, N., Coulomb-Cabagno, G., Traclet, A., & Rascle, O. (2004). Referees' decision making in handball and transgressive behaviors: Influence of stereotypes about gender of players'. *Sex Roles*, *51*, 445–53.

[15] Souchon, N., Cabagno, G., Rascle, O., Traclet, A., Dosseville, F., & Maio, G. R. (2009). Referees' decision making about transgressions: The influence of player at the highest regional level. *Psychology of Women Quarterly*, *33*, 445–52.

[16] Ste-Marie, D., & Lee, T. D. (1991). Prior processing effect on gymnastic judging. *Journal of Experimental Psychology: Learning, Memory, and Cognition, 17,* 126–36.

[17] Ste-Marie, D., & Valiquette, S. M. (1996). Enduring memory-influenced biases in gymnastic judging. *Journal of Experimental Psychology: Learning, Memory, and Cognition, 22,* 1498–502.

[18] Ste-Marie, D. (2003). Memory biases in gymnastic judging: Differential effects of surface feature changes. *Applied Cognitive Psychology, 17,* 733–51.

[19] Boyko, R. H., Boyko, A. R., & Boyko, M. G. (2007). Referee bias contributes to home advantage in English Premiership football. *Journal of Sports Sciences, 25,* 1185–94.

[20] Sutter, M., & Kocher, M. (2004). Favoritism of agents: The case of referees' home bias. *Journal of Economic Psychology, 25,* 461–9.

[21] Nevill, A. M., Balmer, N. J., & Williams, A. M. (2002). The influence of crowd noise and experience upon refereeing decisions in football. *Psychology of Sport and Exercise, 3,* 261–72.

[22] Balmer, N. J., Nevill, A. M., & Lane, A. M. (2005). Do judges enhance home advantage in European championship boxing. *Journal of Sports Sciences, 23,* 409–16.

[23] National Basketball Association (2012). Legends profile: Michael Jordan. http://www.nba.com/history/legends/michael-jordan/index.html (accessed 28 January 2013).

[24] Plessner, H., & Betsch, T. (2001). Sequential effects in important referee decisions: The case of penalties in soccer. *Journal of Sport and Exercise Psychology, 23,* 200–5.

[25] Brand, R., Schmidt, G., & Schneeloch, Y. (2006). Sequential effects in elite basket-ball referees' foul decisions: An experimental study on the concept of game management. *Journal of Sport and Exercise Psychology, 28,* 93–9.

[26] Schwarz, W. (2011). Compensating tendencies in penalty kick decisions of referees in professional football: Evidence from the German Bundesliga 1963–2006. *Journal of Sports Sciences, 29,* 441–7.

[27] Vanden Auweele, Y., Boen, F., De Geest, A., & Feys, J. (2004). Judging bias in synchonized swimming: Open feedback leads to nonperformance-based conformity. *Journal of Sport and Exercise Psychology, 26,* 561–71.

[28] Mussweiler, T. (2003). Comparison processes in social judgment: Mechanisms and consequences. *Psychological Review, 110,* 472–89.

[29] Damisch, L., Mussweiler, T., & Plessner, H. (2006). Olympic medals as fruits of comparison? Assimilation and contrast in sequential judgments. *Journal of Experimental Psychology: Applied, 12,* 166–78.

[30] Schweizer, G., Plessner, H., Kahlert, D., & Brand, R. (2011). A video-based training method for improving soccer referees' intuitive decision-making skills. *Journal of Applied Sport Psychology, 23,* 429–42.

6

INTERACTION AND GAME MANAGEMENT

Game or competition management is a very broad concept that has several sub-components. First it includes *game organisation* – the logistical arrangements of officiating an event from checking the facilities, greeting the athletes and coaches, through to writing match reports. Second there is a decision-making element which extends what we learnt in Chapter 5 and looks at the appropriateness of the decision for the game context, known as *contextual judgement*. Third is the *communication* component, which has a big impact upon the athlete's perceptions of the referee as fair. This chapter will discuss what we know about all three areas, with an emphasis on the official as an interactor, although there will be some elements that also apply to monitors and reactors. Surprisingly, this is an area that has received very little research (though this is expanding). This is due to the fact that the significance of game management in officiating differs between sports. Indeed, a lot of the work draws upon the studies that have been conducted in rugby union where game management is a central task for referees. Sections of this chapter also draw upon our experiences of support work with international referees, while also revealing the links to popular texts and common terminology in sports officiating.

Game organisation

For many officials, preparation for their next appointment begins at least a week beforehand (physical training and preparation may begin much earlier) and, in the case of tournament officiating, preparation can begin months in advance. Often preparation begins with a review of an official's last game, identifying a few key points of emphasis for the future. For some, such as professional referees, there is the luxury of watching recent videos or DVDs of the teams involved in the upcoming contest. Even amateur referees, however, can benefit from a telephone call to the referee who previously officiated the teams to ascertain patterns that occurred during the game. While this information could bias perceptions about certain players or team behaviours (see Chapter 5), it can also be a valuable way of exposing emerging trends in the game. There may well be logistical preparation with the team of co-officials, such as transport/hotel arrangements and organising a time to meet before the game, often as long as two hours before it is due to begin. Checking that the playing facilities are fit for competition, particularly with respect to weather conditions, is sometimes a crucial responsibility. In professional games, this must also account for spectator safety, such as the details of getting to the venue.

This time before the game is the first opportunity to engage with players and coaches, so a balance between adopting a professional approach to pre-game logistics but also showing a human side may stand officials in good stead for maintaining that relationship during the game.

Although game organisation may require some very important decisions to be made, this is a relatively structured process that can often be completed through good preparation and pre-game and post-game routines. However, interactors are also required to develop the much more challenging skills of contextual judgement, where they are expected to adapt their refereeing to the particular characteristics of each game.

Contextual judgement

A referee's knowledge and feel for a game is crucial to applying the spirit of the laws rather than simple adherence to a strict application of the letter of the law.[1] In addition, sports competitions sometimes create unusual situations that demand creative and fair solutions by officials beyond the rulebook (see the example in Box 6.1).

BOX 6.1 MANAGING TOUGH DECISIONS

In February 2012, referee Dave Pearson was forced to call off the France versus Ireland Six Nations game moments before kick-off due to a frozen pitch. Recognising that this would be an unpopular decision and that the organisers, players and fans all wanted the game to go ahead, he felt that player safety was paramount. Fortunately, in this case both coaches backed the referee's decision, but making tough decisions like this is a crucial part of a referee's responsibility.

Because games vary markedly, referees may be required to alter their style of refereeing to suit the particular nuances of the game. In fact, for certain more open invasion games, this judgement may have a greater influence on their decisions than the pursuit of 'robotic consistency' in the application of the rules.[2, 3] Such apparent 'malleability' in the rules may explain, at least in part, why studies in referee decision making[4, 5] have shown that top-class referees are much less than 100 per cent accurate in their application of the rules on a series of snapshot incidents. This influence of contextual judgement appears to be governed by both individual factors – the personal characteristics of the referee in charge such as their refereeing style and philosophy – and game factors that are features of the particular game being officiated (see Box 6.2 for an example of a complex officiating situation in which context was taken into account).

BOX 6.2 A COMPLEX CASE

The 2008 Olympic Medal Race in 49er Sailing was a true nail-biter. The contestants had to face very difficult conditions with wind and waves at the upper limits and every boat capsized at some stage during the race. Two boats even failed to finish inside the time limit. Six crews were in contention for the gold medal and it was the Danes' Jonas Warrer and Martin Ibsen who made this race memorable and created one of those stories that make the Olympics such a special event. Before the race they had a rather comfortable lead and a solid race should have been enough for them to take the victory. On the way to the start, however, they capsized, their mast broke, and their boat was left severely damaged. Quick-thinking, the Danes returned to shore where their coach arranged with the Croatian crew, who did not qualify for the medal race, to borrow their boat. The Danes then raced back to the starting area, under false colours, with only a few seconds to spare and entered the race almost four minutes after the starting signal. They completed the race and came in seventh, giving them enough points to claim gold.

The real drama, however, unfolded after the race. The Spanish crew, who had won the race and therefore won the silver medal, and the Italians, who finished fourth, protested against the result, claiming that the Danes had taken advantage of the situation and that their borrowed replacement boat did not comply with the official requirements. After a long jury hearing until late into the night, the results remained unofficial until another meeting the next morning. The fact that the Danish coach notified the Race Committee of the replacement at the first reasonable opportunity and that the Danish crew presented the replacement boat for inspection immediately after the race led to a dismissal of the protest and consequently to the confirmation of the results. Although the boat did not fulfil all requirements for the medal race – for instance, there was no camera installed and the boat was still equipped with the Croatian flag – the jury decided that the Danes, given the difficult race conditions, did not have an illegal advantage and were declared the winners of the gold medal.

Contextual judgement: individual factors

Refereeing style

Elite referees suggest that you must penalise the clear, obvious and expected infringements (Chris White and Wayne Barnes, elite rugby union referees, personal communication). However, there is some latitude in the rules to enforce them strictly or to allow the players a little more freedom. This is often governed by the particular referee's style or philosophy. There have been many different classifications of refereeing style, including:

- *The dictator*: This style is sometimes referred to as 'robotic refereeing' as these referees apply a strict application of the letter of the law like a schoolmaster. This is often derogatively termed a 'pernickety' or fussy style, although there is anecdotal evidence to suggest that some players prefer it as the clarity of this style reduces the need for players to think about whether their actions will be punished or not. Often, the less players say to these types of officials the better.[6]
- *The teacher*: Here the referee offers a clear understanding of the reasoning behind the decision to educate the players and prevent them from infringing again. These explanations are designed as preventive measures to ensure a clear standard is set and players know when they have overstepped the line. This has also been referred to as the 'judge', who ensures players know how severe the infringement was, letting the punishment fit the crime.
- *Laissez faire style*: This style is where the referee lets the game flow as much as possible and only penalises when a crystal clear infringement has been made.

Practical experiences working with rugby union referees suggests that there may be two other styles, perhaps as a consequence of the complexity of the laws in rugby union[7] creating greater latitude in their application.

- *The 'momentum' referee*: One who favours the attacking team and tries to encourage flowing play in order to quench the spectator's thirst for higher scoring games (M. Mellick, personal communication, 27 March 2013).
- *The 'contest' referee*: One who treats every situation as an independent contest and rewards the dominant 'deserved' team in each situation (M. Mellick, personal communication, 27 March 2013).

As the research is still limited, it is unclear whether these styles are (i) reflections of personality traits; (ii) something more measured, as the referee enacts a role in the 'theatre of sport' (see ideas later in this chapter on *corporate theatre*); or (iii) perhaps a sub-component of one's refereeing philosophy.

Refereeing philosophy

Philosophy can also include things that referees refer to as 'setting out your stall', whereby a referee may begin a game with more of a dictator style in order to keep the players in check, in the belief that it is relatively easier to 'loosen the reins' rather than 'tighten the reins'. Setting standards in such a fashion, however, doesn't seem to be the pattern of elite referees. The elites seem to have the ability (perhaps built upon their experience and confidence) to see what is thrown at them and adjust accordingly. As an International Rugby Board (IRB) referee, Wayne Barnes puts it:

> 'I think it's impossible to set standards. To me this means you're gonna start to referee a way that you're not going to continue, whereas set parameters might be better – this is what's acceptable and this is what isn't.'

Similarly, a former international rugby referee, Chris White, commented on top-flight refereeing as being more akin to a problem-solving exercise than a decision-making task. He suggested that it's about "finding a set of solutions that work for you on the day". This may be a contentious statement amongst many officials whose holy grail is to create 'consistency' in how they apply the rules (laws). However, this statement reflects the idea that referees don't know what they're going to be presented with. Chris says:

> 'You have a set of pictures for how it should look but how what you're confronted with will vary. It's a bit like an electrician who arrives at a house and has to establish the problem? What's broken? What are the clues as to why it's broken? And what do I have in my toolbox to fix the problem? So, on a muddy day you may stand closer, say more at the breakdown (tackle) and allow a little more leniency – so each game is different.'

Perhaps these comments are symptomatic of the complexity of rugby union where there is such latitude in the interpretation of the laws. Accordingly, another former English Premiership referee stated that his goal was to be 'fathomable,' recognising that he has his own style and that, as long as he was consistent within himself, then the players would be able to recognise what would represent legal and illegal play. However, even officials refereeing soccer (the game that FIFA like to refer to as 'the simple game') discuss the idea of consistency within the 90 minutes, recognising that different games require different styles of refereeing.[8]

Material effect

Whilst discussing refereeing style, it would be remiss of us not to discuss the concept of 'material effect' and the referee's ability to adjudicate if infringements have had an impact on the play. This is a clearly established concept that is incorporated into refereeing rulebooks. For example, the International Basketball Federation (FIBA) states:[9]

> The officials should not seek to interrupt the flow of the game unnecessarily in order to penalize incidental personal contact, which does not give the player responsible an advantage nor place his opponent at a disadvantage [p. 50].

This is also an idea that is embraced by practitioners at the top level. Chris White recounts his thoughts during an illegal play in a rugby union tackle:[5]

> I've seen that, it's a penalty, hold on, hold on, it's okay the ball is out – play on. Put your guns in the holster. But you've recognised it and log it for future comment. It's like a suspended sentence [p. 107].

So, it seems that referees apply a *weighting* to their decisions that is influenced by their individual style, their philosophy and also the material effect upon the play. However, research has also investigated within-game factors that influence game management.

Contextual judgement: game factors

In an attempt to develop our understanding of the impact of in-game contextual factors, one study consisted of focus group interviews with members of a rugby union national panel of referees. The referees were asked to review isolated video clips of game decisions and were asked: (i) What might occur around that event (either before or afterwards) that could alter your decision? and (ii) Might you referee this situation differently in different games or for different individuals and, if so, why and in what ways would you modify your decision making and behaviour? Through a process of independent and then collective responses, the two groups of referees (six high potential national panel referees and four full-time international referees) identified five factors that could affect their decisions and then rated how much influence or 'weight' (from 1– 10) each had upon their decisions. The top five characteristics were temper of the game, level of player respect/rapport, position on the pitch, scoreline and time in the game (see Table 6.1).

Temper of the game and level of player respect/rapport

The idea that referees should adapt their decisions to the idiosyncrasies of each game is not new. In fact, FIBA official rules state that, when judging personal contact or violations, referees should consider:[9]

> Consistency in the maintenance of a balance between game control and game flow, having a 'feeling' for what the participants are trying to do and calling what is right for the game [p. 50].

TABLE 6.1 Referees' weightings of the influence of contextual factors on their decisions (1 = no weighting to 10 = very high weighting)[10]

Contextual factor	Mean	SD
Temper of the game	7.60	1.17
Players' respect/rapport	7.10	1.66
Position on the pitch	6.10	2.13
Scoreline	5.90	1.73
Time in the game	5.60	2.22

The appreciation for the tension between creating flow and exerting control seems to be governed by empathy for players[10] and the desire to protect skill. This mindfulness for balance is particularly crucial in open invasion games such as basketball, soccer, handball, rugby league/union, lacrosse, field/ ice hockey, American football and netball, all of which have the potential for open and flowing passages of play. In much the same way as a police officer attempts to prevent crime, the referee in open sports has a similar responsibility: encouraging players to play within the laws so that flow (and spectacle) may be maintained. Thus, a referee may penalise a minor infringement or allow play to develop and manage the situation by being particularly expressive in the condemnation of the player involved to prevent the action from reoccurring. This elasticity in the rules seems to represent good practice yet, in many sports, coaches and the media continue to perpetuate the need for a consistent and consequently unfeeling application of the rules.[11] Later in this chapter we will discuss how research has begun to unravel how elite referees use their game management techniques to send clear messages to players about future encroachments of the rules.

Position on the field, time in the game and scoreline

A post-game 'think aloud protocol', where three referees reviewed their English premiership rugby union games by pausing their game DVD after every tackle incident and verbalising their thoughts at the time, was the first attempt to try to further our understanding of contextual judgement.[5] As well as indicating their thoughts they were asked whether their verbal and non-verbal management of each incident was soft, medium or hard, indicating the strictness of their communication. The majority of tackles were managed with soft responses, but this progressed to a medium response when the field position, time in the game and scoreline became more crucial. Comments from the referees exemplifying this were:

> '[The] defensive player was on the wrong side . . . The ante's moved up. The defensive line has been moved back 20 meters through 2–3 phases, so there's space and potential opening up there. You're moving up the pitch as well and the attack could turn into a try scoring opportunity. There's potentially more interest for the defenders to stop it developing, so my response goes to medium.' (Referee A)

> 'This guy came in from the side. He didn't listen to me . . . Deliberately killing the ball. It was a medium response because greens should've scored here and that's what I was looking at . . . Very hair raising because it's in the red zone. The red zone is an area 10 meters from the try line where the defense will be quite happy to commit the three points for the penalty so that it stops the opposition getting seven points [for a converted try].' (Referee B)

So there seems to be evidence that context not only affects referees' decisions but also their communication to players. The link between the decision and the way in which the situation is managed, such as how the referee convinces others of the appropriateness of that decision or how firmly the referee chastises player behaviour, therefore seems to be an important communication characteristic.[6, 12]

Communication

To date, there has been remarkably little research investigating the crucial area of communication within sports officials. Notably, Mellick and colleagues have looked at decision-communication, emphasising the link between making a decision and selling it to the 'audience'.[13] Recently the audience has been recognised to be very broad in elite refereeing, where the official has been shown to communicate for television commentators and viewers in addition to the players and coaches.[14] Similarly, as described earlier in the chapter, researchers have investigated the nature of referee communications when the penalty for players' transgressions can have a greater impact upon the game (contextual judgement).[15] Such evidence suggests referees' use of 'preventive communication' in order to guide players away from infractions.[15] Currently, researchers in Australia are investigating opinions of referee communication in elite referee managers responsible for developing officials in invasion games (highly interactive sports). This section will highlight these findings, which suggest that these skills are overarched by a clear understanding of the official's role, followed by four related themes including qualities and personality, one-way communication, 'display' skills, situation monitoring and interaction skills.[16]

Referee qualities and personality

Research that has helped to develop our understanding of referee performance includes a study that interviewed 15 select group English Premiership soccer referees.[10] All 15 referees commented on the importance of effective game management as the top characteristic of a skilled official, alongside mental toughness. The referees were then asked about the key components of game management. They identified that communication skills and establishing player and manager respect are central elements. Other components of game management that the referees identified are listed in Table 6.2, indicating the percentage who indicated each.

TABLE 6.2 Most frequently noted characteristics of effective game management[10]

Characteristic of game management	*Percentage of respondents*
Conveying positive body language	66.6%
Building player trust	46.6%
Talk to players and managers	40%
Empathy for players	40%
Build rapport with players and managers	40%
Optimal viewing angle	40%
Awareness of player/manager behaviour	33.3%
Forming relationships	26.6%
Accuracy of big decisions	26.6%
Have banter with players	26.6%

More recently, analysis of ten interviews with national and state level referee development managers in Australia highlighted a range of referee qualities and traits. The positive traits that were used to identify good referees were that these individuals are respectful, professional, empathetic, approachable, decisive, calm, confident, personable and resilient. Negative traits associated with referees included being dictatorial, domineering, over-controlling and officious.[16]

Clearly, refereeing decisions can have an impact on the way referees are perceived, but it appears that effective communication at times can be more important than the decisions themselves. Even when poor decisions are made, if they are communicated effectively they are often received more positively than poorly communicated decisions that may be 100 per cent accurate. In essence, the clarity of explanation that the referee provides can outweigh the accuracy of the decision.[6] Moreover, players rate referees as more fair and correct when they communicate decisions calmly or provide a short interpretation of the decision.[17]

A basic linear model of communication involves a sender, the channel source of information and the receiver.[18] Taking the widely accepted philosophy that the most important part of the communication chain is the receiver – in this case often the player who has contravened the rules – then this is where the referee's focus should be. The thrust of such communication should be to persuade the player that they have infringed the rules in order to secure their acceptance of the sanction. As such, a 'person-centred' approach[19] may be the most effective, with the implication that the same decision may be communicated to two different players in very different ways. This person-centred style is non-directive, where the referee is empathetic to the player's position with unconditional positive regard rather than judgmental and threatening.

One-way communication

Communication skills have been sub-divided into verbal skills (which include the language, paralanguage and delivery) and non-verbal skills. Paralanguage includes things such as volume, articulation, pitch, emphasis and rate, sometimes referred to as the VAPER model. Referees must ensure that each of the VAPER characteristics is set at the appropriate level and recognise that, as they experience stress, each of these is likely to increase so that we speak faster, with greater articulation and a higher pitch, volume and emphasis.

The VAPER model certainly has its uses, but we must not forget that communication is a humanistic activity and breaking it down in a formulaic fashion can sometimes be overly mechanistic and without feeling. For example, imagine having to eject a basketball player who collides with an opponent and falls to the floor. In a rush of blood she kicks out at the player to trip them. By the letter of the law the referee must disqualify the player for unsportsmanlike behaviour. In communicating the sanction, the VAPER model might help the official ensure the message is delivered slowly and with clarity, perhaps something like "I'm really sorry but I'm bound by the rules to disqualify any player who kicks out and trips another player". But if this line is delivered without sincerity or empathy, then the communication may be ineffective. Such times often require the referee to display his/her acting skills, known as impression management.

Non-verbal communication for referees includes the following:

- Facial expressions
- Appearance
- Eye contact
- Proximity
- Haptics
- Orientation
- Body language and posture
- Gestures and signalling
- Use of whistle

Body language is also very important when communicating the 'no-call'. Typically, this is done by an open palm gesture. Although this seems a small intervention, it says: "I've seen it and it doesn't merit a decision". Referees who do not offer such gestures open themselves up to criticism from the players and coaches and the other multiple audiences.

When top national level basketball, rugby union and netball officials have been asked to profile the characteristics of an elite official in their sport, a recurring attribute is *presence*.[20, 21] When we try to think of a sports official with presence, the soccer referee Pierluigi Collina may spring to mind. He had a physically fit body, a strong posture (see Chapter 3) and a look in his eyes that could often say more than his voice.

During flashpoints or critical incidents in games, communication becomes even more critical. Support work with rugby union touch judges has prescribed two short acronyms – RAC and CAC – to guide them on reporting foul play to referees. First, the touch judge must ensure that their body language is Relaxed, Assured and Confident. Then they must portray their message Clearly, Accurately and Concisely (see Figure 6.1 for an illustration of these principles). The Rugby Football Union also had a protocol for reporting the event, beginning with the shirt colour, the shirt numbers of the players involved, followed by a description of what happened in non-litigious language. The open microphone system that is becoming increasingly prevalent in professional sport allows the television audience to hear the assistant referee's voice when reporting foul play via the referee's microphone. The touch judge thus has to be mindful of using appropriate language to help the referee make the correct decision. For example, saying "he stamped on the player's head", an action that is clearly written in law as punishable with a red card and an automatic citing would leave the referee with no option but to send the player off, whereas a phrase such as "unnecessary use of the feet" is both less emotive and would allow the referee to make a judgement based on both officials' interpretations of events.

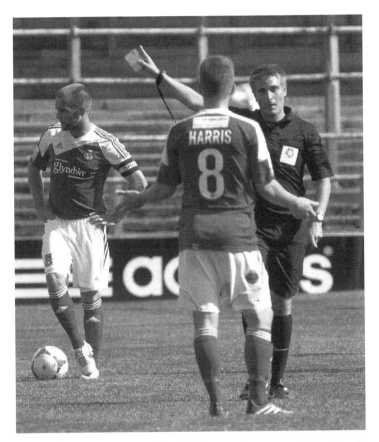

FIGURE 6.1 Referee giving out a red card (photograph courtesy of Les Evans).

Following a decision, a referee must first engage the offender's attention, project confidence in the decision and then foster the perception of a fair and just decision.[14] Knowing which decisions need selling and which will be easily accepted is also a skill that officials develop with experience.

Interaction skills: communication skills versus skilled communication

The exploration of communication skills has usually centred on conflict management skills, as well as the general skill set required for effective officiating. However, recent research reveals that, not only is there a need for specific communication skills such as explaining an interpretation by referring to the rule book but, perhaps more importantly, humanistic judgement skills are also required to allow the referee to get a feel for fluctuations in player temperaments and to develop effective strategies to manage them. This effective interaction has thus been termed 'skilled communication' and can be likened to a 'person-centred' approach to refereeing[19] which relies on effective conflict management skills.

Conflict management

First it is important to recognise that conflict is inevitable in sports officiating. Much of what we are taught about conflict management stems from research on teams of individuals who are trying to work together in a task; however, the very nature of sport means that athletes are competing against each other, so conflict is often inescapable. Nevertheless, officials should recognise that there is a range of styles available to them in order to regulate this conflict and also to manage any conflict that may arise between themselves and the players (see Figure 6.2 for examples of different responses to conflict that illustrate different styles).

Referees who are able to switch in and out of different conflict management styles tend to be those who are most effective at managing conflict. For example, a forceful style may be appropriate when a player has made a hard foul. In contrast, an accommodating style encourages two-way communication and may help to develop a relationship with a player to prevent him from future infringements. It is clear in contrasting these two styles that both may be needed in the one game, by the one referee, for different situations. Thus, reading the situation/person effectively will allow the referee to know when to be forceful and apply the law firmly, but also when to accommodate. This accommodation skill is crucial as it allows the players/coaches to have their say and for both parties (officials and players) to emphasise their differences, but also develop congruency.[22] This is known as the

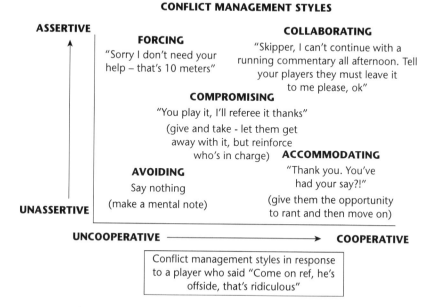

FIGURE 6.2 Kilman's grid with refereeing examples. Adapted from *International Journal of Sport Psychology*, 37, 99–120, Mascarenhas, D. R. D., O'Hare, D., & Plessner, H., The psychological and performance demands of association football refereeing, 2008, with permission from Edizioni Luigi Pozzi.

'voice effect', where people tend to view situations as more fair when they are given an opportunity to express their feelings.[23] Crucially, referees should reflect upon the style that they tend to use as this is the style that they are likely to resort to when the pressure is on, when in fact flexibility of style is needed to ensure that the style is appropriate for the characteristics of the situation encountered. Of course, we note that no matter how good a referee is at managing conflict, there are many situations in which at least one party is unhappy.

Situation monitoring

Building on a cognitive-behavioural approach to understanding human behavior,[24] a helpful tool for referees in understanding communication is the ABC model (see Figure 6.3), which suggests that antecedents lead to certain behaviours and then consequences.[25] For example, a player may miss an open goal, commit a turnover or be on the receiving end of a hard challenge from an opponent (antecedent); the player may then become frustrated and shout at the referee or commit a silly foul (behaviour), and the referee must then penalise the player (consequence).

Referees often see the behaviour but miss the antecedent, or the multiple antecedents. Becoming more fine-tuned to typical antecedents can help referees to manage situations before the behaviour occurs (see Chapters 2 and 3 for discussion of the value of previously competing in the sport).

In order to understand how best to respond to the antecedents, behaviours and consequences of an event, it is helpful to have an appreciation of constructivism theory.[19] This theory of communication suggests that there are three layers to the communication process: social perception, message production and message reception. The theory identifies a backdrop to communication based upon social perceptions. For the players, this backdrop may be the expectation that the referee will be power hungry, over-officious or incompetent (unfortunately this is often the perception of players). For the fans, the expectation may be that the referee will be biased against their team or inconsistent and make crucial mistakes (an idea often perpetrated by scrutiny from media pundits).[26] The message production

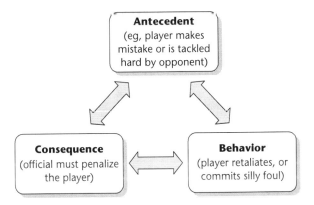

FIGURE 6.3   The ABC model adapted for interactor sports officiating.

phase is where the referee sends the message often both verbally and non-verbally. If we align message production to accommodation theory, then the referee should tailor the message to the recipient. Recent research suggests that, at the top level, the recipients are multiple audiences.[14] For example, the increased use of referee microphones at the top level allows for the official's voice (and often the players' voices too) to be heard by the players, the coaches, the media, the spectators (both in the stadium and at home), as well as the refereeing body who is responsible for making referee appointments/assignments. These different levels have been referred to as micro, meso and macro levels of communication. The micro represents communication with a player (sometimes verbally and often non-verbally); the meso refers to communication directed at all the players on the field; and macro communication is directed to the wider audience that could include the crowd, the media and perhaps the viewing public at home. The way in which referees communicate to this range of audiences has been referred to as *corporate theatre*.[14]

Corporate theatre

A construct that is now used for developing elite referees, corporate theatre is where the referee enacts a role, like a piece of theatre. This is nicely articulated by an international rugby union referee who describes the idea in penalising a player for collapsing a scrum:

> '[You say to them]: "You had a long bind, it's moved to an inside bind, the scrum has collapsed", you haven't even said that he collapsed it. So you've got a get out clause there. So you've told the player what's happened. He can't argue with that. You've told the commentator what happened, who then watches the replay and says "Look he's right. He has changed his bind, the scrum has gone on the floor, good decision referee." The public then hears it and so you're just selling your decisions, like corporate theatre isn't it?'

Such a recounting of the play serves to both justify and explain the referee's decision to all who hear the communication. A similar example occurred at an international rugby union match where the referee penalised a player for interfering with the 'lifter' (the player who has responsibility for lifting a team mate to catch a ball thrown in at height) at a lineout. Rather than just penalising the player and stating "interference with the lifter," the referee took the opportunity to sell himself by stopping the game and calling the player over. Very aware of his multiple audiences, the referee addressed the player: "Remember we talked about this pre-game, you must not interfere with the lifter across the lineout – penalty to blue". So the referee explained the decision, but also told the listeners that he had already pre-warned all the players about such infringements prior to the game, thus portraying himself as both fair and competent. Impression management skills such as these are used to help audiences perceive the referee as competent, dependable and respectable, all of which help to portray the referee as fair.[27] In sum, referees often seem to present themselves in certain ways in order to create an impression, just as a teacher would play 'angry teacher' to get a response from the students without actually feeling the anger.

Summary and conclusion

Although researchers are beginning to investigate the area of game management in officiating, it is clear that it is a large area of work with skills critical to many officials. We have discussed the three components of game management of organisation, contextual judgement and communication. Organisation is the seemingly most straightforward component of game management, which includes responsibility for the general safety of venues. Officiating is an example of a domain that has no shortage of examples of contextual judgement. Sports decision making can thus be argued to make a contribution to understanding decision making in other domains. In contrast, we can apply much of what is known about communication from other domains to help us understand the uniqueness of officiating and particularly refereeing. Moreover, we have discussed the fact that there are multiple refereeing styles. It is unclear if there is a preferred refereeing style, as different players appear to prefer different styles. For example, for some players a robotic style takes away any thinking about the refereeing so they can dedicate their attention to playing. Others may prefer the referee to reward the team who has momentum and advantage and some like to see good attacking play rewarded. Future sports officiating research should explore players' and coaches' preferences for different refereeing styles to see if there is a style that should predominate in certain sports/situations. Also, we hope that research will be directed towards improving our ability to measure refereeing style so that we can develop an appreciation of the weighting that is placed upon referee decisions – for example, if one is more *laissez faire*, or more dictatorial and, indeed, if these labels are helpful measures of effective refereeing style. Hopefully this will help referees to develop familiarity with their own pre-dispositional style and allow them to explore the use of other styles that may be more effective in different situations.

Official's call

Wayne Barnes

Game preparation and organisation

Game management is a crucial part of top-flight officiating and game organisation and preparation form the first part of the process, with many important phases.

Game organisation includes the nuts and bolts of packing my kit, knowing what time I'm leaving the hotel and where the changing room is, etc., all of which are important. However, perhaps more important is my preparation for the contest that's going to take place on the field, which has two elements.

First I will do my homework; 'game prep' is very important for me. In the Premiership we'd generally speak to the referees who have officiated the teams previously to see how the game went. This is not to gain any preconceived ideas, but to see the picture in my head of a player (particularly a front row) getting it right and getting it wrong. It also allows me to prevent some offences before the game begins: a telephone call in the week, a chat with the coach or player beforehand to remind him of what has been agreed or what the law says. This often makes it easier for players to understand their responsibilities. Once I've got a picture as to the context of the upcoming game, I'm also keen to ensure that the team of officials who are working the game are on the same song sheet. So we'll meet beforehand. If it's a European game we'll meet the night before and have a chat over dinner on games and interpretations, showing clips of agreed processes and making sure they are comfortable. This gives us a better chance of working together as a seamless unit. So we'll have an iPad or MacBook, perhaps showing clips of recent games so that they've got the same pictures in their heads that I have – for example, "these are the body positions that I hope to see in the scrum, and this is what I expect of players in the tackle". It's also about reminding ourselves of our agreed protocols. So, if this happens, then the assistant referees know to do this and we're all working together in synergy.

If you're away for three weeks – for example, for a Lions tour of the southern hemisphere – we can all review the game together and improve upon each game, but that's a luxury having the same team of officials for such a block of time. We are trying to do it when we can in the Premiership – with the same two assistant referees – so you're learning from the game before, but it's not always possible.

Then sometime after breakfast (again for a European game) we'll have a pre-match briefing so it gives the assistant referees a chance to reflect and rehearse what they need to do in their own time. It will usually last anything from 10 to 30 minutes, and it gets us all a bit more tuned into the day ahead. Getting things done early allows each member of the officiating team to prepare in their own way.

Second, it's important to get the coaches on board. Developing a relationship with clubs/coaches is an ongoing process and involves visits to Premiership clubs throughout the season to brief them on law interpretations and points of emphasis. However, importantly, this is reinforced in the build-up to the game. During the week prior to an international fixture I'll speak to both coaches and reinforce what certain laws say and what has been agreed, so that on the game day there are no surprises. For international games, it's almost common practice now to meet the coach one or two days before and to suggest "this is what I expect" and "these are areas that I will emphasise". It's about talking through my expectations of responsibilities and making sure the players know what's expected of them and their expectations of me. It could be me contacting the coach or the coach contacting me, but it will invariably happen. Some will have pre-prepared clips and ask: "Do you think this is okay and what about this? How will you manage this sort of situation and what if the opposition do this, will we be allowed to do this?" etc. It's just their way of getting clarity on what's expected of them – which works well. Other coaches will come in and ask: "What will we do to help you?", which also works.

Then, on game day I'll meet with just the players, which is just a reminder of what we spoke about with their coach. You meet the front row players, the scrum-half and then the captain during the toss. This will take place sometime in the two hours before kick-off; sometimes the time will be prearranged and other times not, but the players always know that it will happen at some point. At this point it's largely just about reinforcement of what they already know. There's rarely a great deal of detailed discussion, but often they'll have questions such as: "What's your take on this and this?" – and it works too – no surprises – just reminders. I'll see both teams separately, which I guess helps free-flowing discussion.

Postponing games

I was standing next to Dave Pearson when the France versus Ireland game was called off, as mentioned in the chapter. We were in constant discussion with the coaches, getting their views and as much information from them as possible. It's not purely the referee's decision. It's important to consult with the groundsmen, the players and the coaches – they're all involved in the decision.

Any postponement when teams disagree is difficult as you become the sole arbiter. Only once have I said a pitch was playable when one of the teams said it was not. The game went ahead, thankfully without issue or injury. It was a waterlogged pitch, so I had to ensure I listened to the coaches' concerns and used all of the available resources to deal with the concerns (namely getting the water off) and, crucially, explaining throughout what I was doing. TV was also present, so you have to manage the media's expectations too. We had to move the kick-off from 8.00pm to 8.30pm so you don't then antagonise a stakeholder. If you've got one coach saying it's fit to play, and another saying it's not, your instinct is to err on the side of player safety. Often you'll also have conversations in the week beforehand to prevent the long drive for the away team. A former referee coach of mine used to recount a game he did between two of the top teams (Gloucester versus Leicester), and he'd say: "If there's a former English international player and an ex-British Lion's player (the two coaches) saying that it's unfit, then you'd be stupid to disagree or not listen to them". You have to err on the side of caution, but it is really a collaborative decision.

Contextual judgement and material effect

Players dictate the How of a game. If a team wants to play slow rugby where they pick and drive, reset (slowly pick up the ball and work it forwards), get your forwards out, we cannot do much. We can prevent a team illegally slowing opposition ball, we can try and prevent teams trying to stop a team's flow by going down injured, but we are limited in what we can do. What is important is that we understand this context (contextual judgement) and referee material effect, or the majority of games will be constantly stopped. The best example is when the winger is offside twenty meters away from the ruck (where the ball is) and the attacking scrum-half is only ever going to go in the opposite direction to the winger. His whole team is going this way and no one even looks to the other side. How can that winger have an effect on the game? By the letter of the law it should be penalised, but clearly it has had no impact upon the game so we continue, allowing some flow. Similarly, the defender who oversteps the offside line but goes back when asked may not need to be penalised if he doesn't gain an advantage from doing so.

It's a bit like preventive refereeing, but to me that means stopping something *before* it has happened. If a player has already illegally slowed down an attack and you say "now let go", we are condoning that action. Preventing is saying "don't go in there" – as a player looks to illegally go into the side of a maul, or "clear release" as the tackle is about to be completed and you sense a player may not clearly release.

Refereeing style

Players and coaches need to know what is acceptable – from "Will the referee allow us to speak to him today?" to "Can we fall the wrong side in the tackle?" By being hard on something in the first five minutes and then not following through until the 79th minute, we can be accused of being inconsistent. If, however, we say this is what is acceptable in minute one and in minute 79, it is difficult to say we are inconsistent. I prefer to think of it as setting parameters of acceptability rather than setting standards.

You want to be able to explain decisions when required (the teacher) but need to be strict with players if they are trying to take advantage of that. So, if I've penalised a team and they say "Ref, can we talk about that decision now?" just as the opposition are already trying to take their penalty quickly, you can see that they're just trying to slow the penalty taker down so that they can get all their team back onside. Sometimes you have to be firm. I also want to give the benefit of doubt to teams going forward (momentum) but also reward a defender who wins a contest and deserves reward. My thoughts on what the players want in terms of style, is just ensuring that they know what to expect of you. Whether that is not being able to talk to you or being approachable, as long as you don't flit between one style and the other without reason.

There's definitely an element of the dictator style sometimes too – for example: "Now isn't the right time to talk – you've just given away a penalty". I'm not going to engage now. You dictate things on your terms. But then you have to be collaborative with players as I may be refereeing the same player next week. I will want to go and find him straight away after the game. Similarly, within the game, at the next stoppage you'll maybe give him a chance to have his rant because you've got to work with him for the time left in the game.

I think we'd all want to be a *laissez faire* type of referee but you've got to have parameters. I think there are definitely aspects when you become a momentum referee, where you only penalise the clear and obvious so, if you have any doubt, you let things go. That automatically means it goes in favour of the attacking team because they've got the ball. And there are times where you become a contest referee as you also have to look at each event so, to get the ball back, the defence has to do something that merits it. All the styles tie into each other. So I think I referee a mixture of different styles depending upon the situations, but I think the players are aware of referees' different styles. It would be naïve to think they weren't. They know the referees they can talk to and what to expect from each. Internationally, teams will prepare areas where they need to adhere a bit more to the law for some officials than for others. So, for example, they'll be aware that "we can have more of a contest with this referee whereas with this guy we need to be a bit more adherent".

In the past, teams have got upset when a referee has been changed the day before a game (usually down to injury) because it may slightly alter the team's approach to certain situations, but it's the same for us as referees. We may prepare for a game where a player has suddenly got injured and all your homework on that player is wasted. That's not to say our preparation involves predicting what players will do, but we might imagine certain scenarios and think about how we would manage them. If it's a new player, then it's more likely that there'll be some surprises thrown in and obviously we don't want too many of those. So it works both ways.

Contextual factors

Of the contextual factors listed, temper of game would be most influential, but it is rare that it would be a factor – for example, after a large fight one of the most influential factors would be temper, but this is rare. Because the fights are rare – more so these days with video citing. Then the position on the pitch is important because you're more aware of quick and slow ball. The defending team acts differently in their own 22 (the line near to their own goal line when they can't afford for a player to break the defensive line) whereas maybe on the halfway line it's less important. In the attacking 22, teams on the front foot and slowing have more of an effect. But a high tackle on the defensive 22 metre line, the halfway line or on the attacking 22 metre line is a high tackle regardless. Only certain offences are affected by contextual factors.

At the professional level you can't say that the scoreline or the time in the game is going to make you be more lenient or indeed stricter. However, if I'm refereeing a local club's third team game, then enjoyment is part of it. It kind of comes down to your refereeing philosophy. At the community level I'm less tied to a strict application of the law so I can loosen the reins a little to allow a little more flow to the game. For example, in the professional game, if the match was very one-sided you would have an issue if you let things go a little more whereas at an under thirteen's game, I would think it would be good game management to allow the losing team a little more leniency because, philosophically, your responsibility is also to help the development of those players. The only thing that may change at the professional level is perhaps the length of advantage that you play if the scoreline is tight at the end of the game. If a team is losing by two points with thirty seconds to play and the team ahead infringes within kickable distance, then the only real advantage to a team is to have a shot at goal. A poor advantage may lead to an 'advantage over' call and a team not having the opportunity to win the game.

The key for top flight officiating is accuracy (as shown in Table 6.2), not just of big decisions but across the game. Forming relationships and building rapport and trust are also really important. This then means that players are less likely to 'infringe'. I guess they are as likely to breach the laws as much as they believe in your ability to catch them, which is probably why it is harder when you start off at Premiership or international level. If the players don't know you, they may think "let's put a bit more pressure on this guy", whereas I know if I was refereeing at a Premiership club where I've been officiating for years (e.g., London Wasps) they'd be more likely to think "we know what the boundaries are already so we don't need to test them".

Models to support good game management

Game management is really important, but I don't think at the top level there's really room for covering up a poor decision with good communication or selling it. It's more likely that, when you've made a poor decision and you've seen it on the big screen and then said to a player: "Sorry mate, I think I got that wrong", it's not about getting away with it, it's about accepting you made the best decision with the view you had at the time, then building bridges with the player who may be grumpy. And the way you communicate with players is probably a mixture of styles as presented in Kilman's grid, except forcing – that would probably just escalate the issue. I would hope that my preferred style would be collaborating, and that's why you do all the work pre-match. Some referees may want to take charge and show their authority, but are you ever in charge as a referee? I don't' think so. The players are in charge of what happens in the game. You just have to make a decision upon what's presented to you. It's more about what they do and what you see. If everyone's aiming for the same outcomes (i.e., working within the same framework), it makes it a lot easier. I might get things wrong because I got the picture wrong (e.g., I was standing in the wrong place or my attention was diverted because of this player's actions), but not because my philosophy is different.

I don't think there is ever a time when you would avoid when you've made a bad decision – avoiding and not listening to the players, no. A player may say something to you in the wrong way or at the wrong time, but I wouldn't avoid when I've made a bad decision. That would be the worst time to avoid. First, you've got to realise that the decision is wrong, which could come from feedback from the players. You'd ask yourself: "Have I missed something?" and perhaps say: "Sorry fellas, I didn't see it". I might have a couple per game at the most, but any more and you start to lose your credibility.

The ABC model is also a helpful tool. Being aware of the antecedents, particularly with foul play, is essential for teams believing that you are treating them fairly. For example, I refereed Northampton versus Worcester in the 2013/14 season and awarded a red card to a Worcester player. If I had just red carded the punch, then

Worcester would have felt hard done by as it was a Northampton player who had been the cause of the punch by holding on to the Worcester player's shirt. By also giving a yellow card to the Northampton player, you keep the trust of Worcester and the players feel they are treated equally.

I think the comments and tools presented in this chapter can be really helpful. They make me ask: "Why do I behave in a certain way on the pitch?" and, more importantly: "How can I do things better?" You can't get away with being too forceful or too loud – it's no good telling people to stop shouting by shouting at them. So these things help to focus your mind a little and make you think about the sort of referee you want to be, and when you behave in certain ways they often provide clues as to why.

References

[1] Askins, L., Carter, T., & Wood, M. (1981). Rule enforcement in a public setting: the case for basketball officiating. *Qualitative Sociology, 4,* 87–101.

[2] Mascarenhas, D. R. D., Collins, D., Mortimer, P., & Morris, R.L. (2005). A naturalistic approach to training coherent decision-making in rugby union referees. *The Sport Psychologist, 19,* 131–47.

[3] Stern, J. (2002). Evaluating officiating performance. *Referee, 27,* 63.

[4] Fuller C.W., Junge, A., & Dvorak, J. (2004). An assessment of football referees decisions in incidents leading to player injuries. *American Journal of Sports Medicine, 32*(Suppl. 1), 17–22.

[5] Mascarenhas, D. R. D. (2005). Helping the man in the middle: Assessing and training referee performance. Unpublished doctoral thesis. Edinburgh: The University of Edinburgh.

[6] Simmons P. (2008). Justice, culture and football referee communication. Paper presented to the I-Come International Communication and Media Conference. University Utara, Kuala Lumpur, Malaysia.

[7] Ackford, P. (2003). Ring of confidence from the whistle blowers. *The Sunday Telegraph,* 16 March, p. 11.

[8] Bennett, S. (2003). Enhanced management skills. *Presentation at the Best of British Rugby League National Coaching Conference to the Super League Referees,* Bolton, UK, 8 November.

[9] International Basketball Federation (FIBA). (2012). *Official basketball rules 2012: As approved by FIBA Central Board.* Rio de Janeiro, Brazil: FIBA.

[10] Slack, L., Maynard, I., Butt, J., and Olusoga, P. (2013). Factors underpinning elite sport officiating: Perceptions of English Premier League referees. *Journal of Applied Sport Psychology, 25,* 298–315.

[11] British Broadcasting Corporation (BBC). (2012). Bolton boss Owen Coyle 'craves' refereeing consistency. http://www.bbc.co.uk/sport/0/football/16395310 (accessed 28 March 2013).

[12] Askins, R. (1987). Common myths about officiating. *Referee, 26,* 44–7.

[13] Mellick, M. C., Bull, P. E., Laugharne, E. J., & Fleming, S. (2005). Identifying best practice for referee decision communication in association and rugby union football: A microanalytic approach. *Football Studies, 8,* 42–57.

[14] Cunningham, I., Mellick, M., Mascarenhas D. R. D., & Fleming, S. (2012). Decision making and decision communication in elite rugby union referees. *Sport and Exercise Psychology Review, 18,* 19–30.

[15] Mascarenhas, D. R. D., Collins, D., & Mortimer, P. (2005b). Elite refereeing performance: Developing a model for sport science support. *The Sport Psychologist, 19*, 364–79.

[16] Cunningham, I., Simmons, P., Mascarenhas D. R. D., & Redhead, S. (2014). Skilled Interaction: Concepts of communication and player management in the development of sports officials. *International Journal of Sport Communication, 7*(2), 166–187.

[17] Simmons, P. (2010). Communicative displays as fairness heuristics: Strategic football referee communication. *Australian Journal of Communication, 37*, 75–94.

[18] Shannon, C. E., & Weaver, W. (1949). *The mathematical theory of communication.* Urbana, Illinois: University of Illinois Press.

[19] Burleson, B.R. (2007). Constructivism: A general theory of communication skill. In B. B. Whaley, & W. Samter (Eds). *Explaining communication: Contemporary theories and exemplars* (pp. 105–28). Mahwah, NJ: Lawrence Erlbaum Associates.

[20] Mascarenhas, D. R. D. The Psychology of Refereeing. Workshop for Basketball Scotland's National League Referees, Dundee, Scotland, September 2004.

[21] Mascarenhas, D. R. D. The Psychology of Officiating. Southland NZFU Referees' Meeting, Southland, New Zealand, April 2006.

[22] Giles, H., & Ogay, T. (2007). Communication accommodation theory. In B. B. Whaley, & W. Samter (Eds). *Explaining communication: Contemporary theories and exemplars* (pp. 293–310). Mahwah, NJ: Lawrence Erlbaum Associates.

[23] Shapiro, D. L. & Brett, J. M. (2005). What is the role of control in organizational justice? In J. Greenberg & J. A. Colquitt (Eds). *Handbook of organizational justice* (pp. 155–77). New Jersey: Lawrence Erlbaum.

[24] Meichenbaum, D. (1977). *Cognitive behavior modification: An integrative approach.* New York: Harper & Row.

[25] Miltenberger, R. G. (2008). *Behavior modification: principles and procedure, 4th Edition.* Belmont, California: Thomson Wadsworth.

[26] Colwell, S. (2004). Elite level refereeing in men's football: A developmental sociological account. Thesis submitted for the degree of Doctor of Philosophy at the University of Leicester.

[27] Simmons, P. (2011). Competent, dependable and respectful: Football refereeing as a model for communicating fairness. *Ethical Space: The International Journal of Communication Ethics, 8*, 33–42.

7

PSYCHOLOGICAL DEMANDS AND SKILLS

Demands of officiating

In addition to the demands of officiating reviewed in Chapter 2, sports officials need to have a unique blend of self-confidence (sometimes projected self-confidence) in order to sell decisions to players, together with a commitment to self-analysis and self-development through the reflective practice process.[1] At the top level they often have to contend with the spotlight of scrutiny from multiple audiences including the players and coaches, television commentators and, of course, the partisan fans. Yet, top referees appear to be open and honest enough to recognise their mistakes and review them at the right time (often through post-game reflections/debriefs and conversations with players, coaches and peers), as well as having the ability to project an image of fortitude and honesty, earning respect from the players/athletes around them.[2]

Although self-confidence and self-critique may appear to be quite dissonant characteristics, they are actually characteristics that we see exhibited by top-flight performers (coaches, athletes, business professionals, airline pilots, surgeons, for example) in a range of situations. The ability to embrace continual critical analysis of one's performance can take tremendous strength of character, which is particularly important for high profile officials who have to contend with negative media attention.

Motivations

We have limited research evidence on referees' motivations to become involved in officiating (see Chapter 2 for a discussion of what we do know) though, anecdotally at least, in the past many have sustained injuries that have prevented them from playing, turning them towards officiating (this appears to be a smaller percentage of interactor officials nowadays, however, as an athletic body image seems to be increasingly important to officiate at the top level). Many referees have come from the domain of education, often as physical education teachers, as well as policing and law (e.g., ex-lawyers). Regardless of the career domain, the vast majority are ex-athletes in the sport they officiate. At the extreme end of this is the recent example of ex-rugby union player Glen Jackson (Saracens, Premiership fly-half) who was fast tracked through the pathway to become a referee. This process led him to become an assistant referee for an international game between Australia and New Zealand within a year of his retirement and, soon after this, to an assignment as the match referee for England versus Fiji after retiring from playing only 24 months previously.

Regardless of pathways, what we do know about officials' motivations is that soccer referees appear to be driven by their devotion to the sport.[1] Players' and coaches' perceptions are often very different, perceiving officials to be driven by power and prestige.

Personality of officials

Interestingly, there still appear to be large differences of opinion between fans, players and even officials themselves on the perceptions of officials' personality types. Athletes and fans rate officials significantly higher than officials rate themselves on expressiveness of emotionality (neuroticism). The athletes and fans also rate officials much lower on extraversion, openness, agreeableness and conscientiousness than officials rate themselves. In fact, an investigation into volleyball, ice hockey and wrestling officials showed that fans and players consistently provided less favourable evaluations of all personality domains than the referees' own self-report ratings.[3] However, it is unclear how much these opinions are self-generated and how much they are perpetuated by the media's portrayal of officials.

Psychological characteristics and skills

Sports officials require a core set of psychological skills and characteristics in much the same way as any elite performer.[4] They must plan their time, create opportunities for physical and mental training, peak for games and develop strategies and systems for reviewing their performance. Crucially, sports officials must not only possess the psychological *characteristics* to allow them to learn and develop their potential, but they must also have a range of psychological *skills* to enable them to perform on match days, when they may be under intense pressure.

Seminal research into Olympic sports performers and golfers in the 1980s showed a range of psychological characteristics that elite athletes possess.[5, 6] Since then, interviews with such performers revealed top athletes to show high levels of commitment, controllable imagery, greater levels of concentration and widespread use of goal setting[7] and social support networks.[8] Unfortunately, to date there is limited evidence on the psychological characteristics required of elite sports officials. Nevertheless, taking the view that elite officials have similar demands to elite athletes, there are a number of prerequisite characteristics that are required in order for officials to realise their potential on the pathway to excellence.[9, 10]

Therefore, this chapter will comprise two sections. The first will explain the key psychological *characteristics* for sports officials:

- Commitment, planning and organisation
- Self-awareness/analysis and critical appraisal
- Distraction/arousal control and clear and present tense focus
- Realistic performance evaluation
- Robust self-belief (this could very easily be linked to self-awareness)
- Passion and joy

With these skills in mind, it is worth noting that mentally tough officials would have the natural or developed psychological edge that enables them to: generally, cope better than others with the many demands (competition, training, lifestyle) that sport places on a performer; specifically, be more consistent and better than peers in remaining determined, focused, confident and in control under pressure.[11]

The second section will describe some of the core psychological *skills* required that can be used to help develop these characteristics:

- Pre-event routines
- Critical self-reflection through pre- and post-game briefings and reviews
- Quality practice
- Self-talk: cue words and triggers (visual and physical)
- Imagery and scenario playing
- Performance planning

In addition we will look at strategies for building self-confidence (interlinked with some of these ideas above) and also the role of the national governing body to support officials through peer and mentor support. Throughout we will highlight what we know from research as well as providing practical examples to show how top officials use these skills to enhance their officiating.

The psychological characteristics of excellence (PCE)

Commitment, planning and organisational skills

Most elite sports officials are older than elite athletes and, whilst some sports offer pathways for full-time officials, the vast majority are part-time. Thus balancing work, family and lifestyle pressures with one's officiating development is a common challenge as most have professional jobs too. For those officials who are still in full-time employment and refereeing part-time, time management is a crucial attribute to ensure that sufficient time can be allocated to self/video-reflection and peer reviews and, in the case of interactor referees, for fitness training. Developing good personal management and regular conversations with other officials and mentors can also create an advantage for officials in coping with likely game situations.

Self-awareness/analysis and critical appraisal

A commitment to self-development and understanding of the self is crucial. There are many different styles to officiating. As discussed by Chris White (see Official's Call later in this chapter), refereeing in rugby union is a process of " . . . finding a set of solutions that work for you on the day". While this may be a contentious explanation of elite officiating, given that it implies that there is a range of ways of refereeing a game rather than robotically applying a set of rules consistently, it is provided by an elite rugby union referee who has refereed over fifty international games (including a World Cup semi-final). The ability to self-reflect upon the decisions that have been made, how they have been communicated and the positioning during the game is a prerequisite for top sports officials. They will review DVDs of their games and reflect upon their decisions and actions, exploring alternative solutions that they can utilise in their next game.

Distraction/arousal control and clear and present tense focus

Arguably the most important psychological skill for an official is to maintain concentration, particularly after a decision error or player conflict. In addition, officials must also deal with the pressure that the 'spotlight' often shines upon them. The best way to describe the effects of pressure upon officiating performance is perhaps through attentional control theory (ACT)[12] because it relates to both anxiety and concentration, which collectively are most likely to have the biggest impact upon officiating performance (see also Chapter 4).

Particularly pertinent to the interactor official, ACT suggests that there are two types of attentional styles: stimulus-driven or goal-directed. The stimulus-driven style, which is also described as bottom-up processing, concerns sensory cues in the environment such as adjudicating whether or not a player is offside. The goal-directed style, known as the top-down approach, encourages individuals to direct their attention to goals and future expectations, which might include such things as trying to allow a game to flow, perhaps by applying an advantage rule, or planning how to manage a player's frustrations during a stoppage in play. ACT proposes that, under normal (non-stressful) situations, individuals are able to easily switch their processing to the style that best fits the situation they are in, so they can easily interchange between top-down and bottom-up processing. Unfortunately, increases in anxiety disrupt the ability to switch easily between these two styles and emphasise the stimulus-driven style at the expense of goal-directed attention. As such, because of this increased activity in sensory perceptions (attention drawn to what is in front an individual), anxious referees are much more likely to be distracted by threatening cues, such as angry or upset players, rather than officiating the play (see Chapters 4 and 5 for information about the relevance of picking up appropriate cues). The message for aspiring sports officials is to avoid this anxiety inducing working memory overload to ensure that they can allocate attention flexibly to fit the situational requirements. In the short term this is very challenging but, in the long term, there are a number of intervention strategies that can alleviate match day pressures.

A programme of stress exposure training,[13] where officials are systematically exposed to demands that exceed those that they will experience on match day, can be an effective training aid to help develop the skills necessary to deal with increased attentional demands (see Box 7.1). Another strategy that has been used very effectively for air traffic control trainees is 'above real-time' training, which subjects trainees to images that move up to 2× faster than they are likely to experience on the job. This method has been used successfully in sport,[14–16] where experts who were exposed to 1.5× normal speed not only improved their accuracy post-test but also became better at high speed situations than they were at normal speed, leading us to believe that they relied on automatic decision processes. Consequently, it seems that video-based Above Real-Time Training (ARTT) may be an effective tool to inoculate referees to increased task demands, allowing them to perform with greater ease, thus saving more processing space for other on-task demands (see Box 7.1) such as recognising a team's defensive strategy and allowing a referee to help anticipate where the play will go (for further discussion see Chapters 4 and 5). Presently there is no research on the effects of ARTT for sports officials. An ARTT intervention may provide invaluable training for officials, however, particularly those stepping up to the next performance level where things happen much more quickly than the referee may be used to.

BOX 7.1 THE GUINNESS PRINCIPLE

Our working memory has a limited storage capacity.[28] We can think of this capacity as a pint glass, and the liquid within as Guinness.[29] The Guinness is made up of 'black stuff' (attention allocated towards performance), and 'white stuff' – the froth (attention allocated towards distracting thoughts and worry).

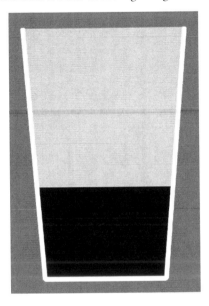

(continued)

(continued)

During a 'comfortable game' (perhaps a youth game) where players are respectful, referees probably have lots of experiences of successful refereeing (see image above). At these sorts of games they will only have about a third of a pint of Guinness (black stuff) with very little froth and lots of free mental processing space to allocate wherever they choose; perhaps joking with the players or coaching them to develop their understanding of the rules.

During a high-pressure game, there may be extra factors competing for the official's attention such as perhaps an abusive fan at the venue or where the game is a lot quicker and they miss one decision then another and another and they find themselves trying to catch-up and make a call while also trying to manage the players' increased frustrations. Here, the Guinness glass is very full of black stuff (a great deal of performance-related processing is required) but there may also be a great deal of white stuff, such as a fan screaming obscenities (external distractions), or the referee's own internal voice saying "s★★t I missed that call, quick call something" (internal distractions). Although it hasn't been empirically tested through scientific study, it seems likely that most distractions eventually manifest as internal distractions. So, as with the abusive fan example above, it is how the individual referee deals with it internally that matters. Whether the referee is able to ignore or manage the distraction or dwell on it (ruminate) will affect how full the glass becomes. Those referees who tend to ruminate are more likely to experience an over flowing glass (see image below) and what psychologists often term 'choking'. To come back from a choking situation is very difficult, thus it is much better to have strategies in place to prevent them in the first place.

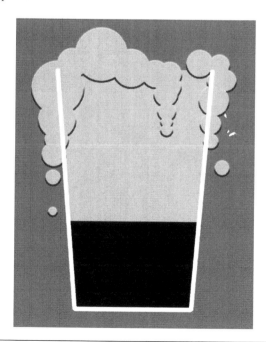

The key to long-term prevention of choking and lapses of concentration during performance is for the official to reduce the amount of processing space (black stuff) required for performance.

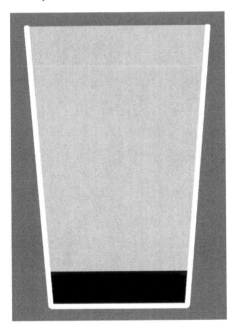

This is achieved by increasing skill level and thus automatizing the officiating process. Automatization can be done through stress exposure training (also known as stress inoculation training) over a period of time where the referee is exposed to increased task demands in a safe environment where s/he can develop the skills to cope with the increased pressure. The pressure can be simulated through fatiguing the referee before asking them to respond to a situation, role-playing in front of their peers or with a camera in their face, or with simulations of visual or audible distractions. This is the same principle used in many domains, including training horses for police work. The assumption is that referees will then learn how to develop self-talk cue-words and triggers to help direct attention appropriately (as described later in this chapter). (Images courtesy of Mark Sheeky.)

Realistic performance evaluation

Players and coaches are often inadequate judges of an official's performance. As a consequence, the high-performance official needs to find a realistic approach to assessing his or her performance. The vast majority of officials will not have the luxury of having an assessor or a coach to provide feedback to them, so video review – and, where possible, peer consultation – can provide a valuable alternative. Honesty in coping with a 'blown call' is often advocated as the best response to officiating errors, and embracing the learning opportunity presented by such mistakes – big or small – is essential.

Robust self-belief

Robust self-belief is crucial for top performance. The research of Albert Bandura[17, 18] suggests that there is no better source of confidence than previous success. Mastery experiences serve to raise efficacy expectations and continual failure lowers efficacy expectations. Félix Guillén and Deborah Feltz introduced the label 'refficacy'[19] to describe referee self-efficacy, which they propose includes mastery experience, referee knowledge/education, support from others, physical and mental preparedness, environmental comfort and perceived anxiety. Although in its infancy, their model, which is largely theoretically driven, seems to provide a valuable starting point for investigation into referee confidence.

Passion and joy

While not strictly a psychological characteristic embedded in research evidence, passion and joy underpin many of the other characteristics. If an official is lacking passion for what they do, it is very difficult to remain motivated and excel. Officials must therefore enjoy their role and what they are doing. As well as the previously emphasised importance of being self-critical, it helps if officials have a sense of humour about their performance and do not take themselves too seriously. An investigation by Philippe and colleagues[4] showed that, from their sample of 90 of the top French soccer referees, every single referee reported that they were passionate about refereeing.

Psychological skills

As mentioned, this section examines the skills that officials can use in order to develop the PCE and will provide practical examples to help the developing official adapt these ideas into their performance.

Pre-event routines

Preparation is everything for the sports official. In fact, some governing bodies emphasise the quality of preparation above all else at the international level, believing that a well-prepared official will make good decisions. In preparing for an upcoming game or competition, committed officials report that they 'do their homework' by taking time to call the referees who last officiated the teams involved. This ensures that the official is aware of any issues that arose previously, which may arise again. Should similar events transpire again, the official is less likely to be surprised and has given himself/herself the opportunity to prepare an appropriate response.

Critical self-reflection through pre- and post-game briefings and reviews

Pre-game briefings are an excellent opportunity to set a tone of professionalism amongst the team of officials. Bringing 'homework', as described above, and having a checklist of points of emphasis, areas of responsibility and procedural protocols are often used as preparation for an officiating team's performance. This also provides a foundation for improved communication between officials (see Chapter 6 for more on this topic). Such professionalism should extend to greeting the coaches. This probably sounds like a very rudimentary procedure, but often at the amateur level referees do not take the time to introduce themselves to the coach and find out the coach's name. Referees who show knowledge of a team and an interest in their performance generally (e.g., "How is your season progressing") create an opportunity to develop rapport with the coach and create a respectful relationship. This facilitates later communication and interaction, particularly if conflict arises. Similarly, referees should use the time between periods of play to confer and discuss issues arising in the game. This can be great preventive refereeing and also helps to ensure that the team are united.

In addition to pre-game briefings and preparation, the development of officials is aided by conducting reflective post-performance analyses. This analysis should involve the entire officiating team and provides a great opportunity to discuss decisions and analyse what went well and what did not go well. If a flashpoint (critical conflict or fight) occurred in the game which requires a report, memory decay suggests that post-performance is the best time to maximise accurate recall. The report should be written up when it is fresh in the referee's mind but, if he/she is still emotionally angry or uptight about the incident, it may be best to make notes to elaborate on later without the emotional baggage that he/she may be carrying. Once the report has been drafted it is good practice to take a break and then to re-read what has been written with a fresh pair of eyes.

In addition to reflection on the performance of the officiating team, each official is advised to reflect upon their own individual performance, perhaps with the assistance of a coach or mentor and, where possible, video review. The four cornerstones model of refereeing[20] provides an excellent template for reflecting upon performance. Specifically, a proposed method is for officials to write a few lines of reflection and evaluation of their performance in each of the following five areas: law application; contextual judgement; personality and game management; fitness and positioning; and psychological characteristics.

Quality practice

Given that a large body of research suggests that expertise in the sporting environment requires 10,000 hours of deliberate practice to master,[21, 22] if an official's match experience lasts approximately 90 minutes, this purely experiential approach would equate to approximately 7,000 matches – the equivalent of refereeing one game per day for 35 years, assuming a season is 200 days long. As a consequence, referees are challenged with finding other meaningful environments to conduct practice. Clearly there is some transfer of knowledge that may emerge from referees watching games, but also from participating as players. It is thus suggested that referees suffer from performing in a practice-poor domain, and must look for knowledge transfer where possible, including reading, study and training courses.

Self-talk: cue words and triggers (visual and physical)

A common technique to avoid the choking and distraction mentioned previously is 'parking'.[23] This technique involves mentally setting aside distractions for later processing to prevent the suboptimal use of resources described earlier. 'Parking' decision errors or poor management of players is a characteristic that requires practice. Research suggests that higher level officials in basketball use more self-talk than lower level referees. What we know from clinical psychology is that cognitive restructuring can be used to prevent people from dwelling on negative thoughts.[24] This involves stopping the negative thought with a phrase as simple as 'stop', then using a positive replacement phrase such as 'focus on the defender', perhaps coupled with a trigger (e.g., placing the whistle in the mouth).

Imagery and scenario playing

Just as athletes use imagery to help prepare themselves for what they are about to encounter in the performance environment, officials often use imagery in order to plan for scenarios that are likely to occur. This planning may be informed by the pre-performance preparation mentioned previously, in which officials obtain information on previous performances. The use of imagery to play out possible scenarios allows officials to develop action plans for the prevention and management of conflict with players, or of expected deceptive play, which pushes the boundaries of the rules or laws of the sport. The importance and role of scenario playing is underscored by the comments of an elite rugby union referee:

> 'I think role play can form an important part in this as well because I know in the past we've done role plays on dealing with foul play situations and it is rehearsal and you can see some of these guys who are dead confident and when your TV's on it's just like (gesturing giving a card in a confident manner) and it has to come back to rehearsal. You have to train your mind as to what you want to say.' (International rugby union referee)

Performance planning

Although referee bodies are constantly challenged with developing and retaining high quality sports officials (see Chapters 2 and 9), there is inevitably considerable competition for those wishing to make it to the very top level. A commitment to goal setting to encourage development in all the requisite skills will undoubtedly help the aspiring official to progress towards her/his target. Goals have been shown to direct attention both cognitively and behaviourally,[25] to increase persistence[26] and also to help people develop strategies in order to achieve them.[27]

Goals are categorised into process goals, performance goals and outcome goals. Process goals highlight the activities and tasks in which one should engage in order to reach the performance goal – for example, "I will memorise the offside law in soccer by next week". Performance goals focus on improvements relative to one's own performance – for example, "I will always stay ahead of the ball or keep up with play by anticipating the movement of the ball". Finally, outcome goals are less controllable as they focus on results – for example, "I will get appointed to officiate one First Division game before the end of the season". Most research suggests that outcome goals serve to enhance motivation whereas process goals provide more direction and actions to attain outcomes.

The simple principle that is frequently used in goal setting is the acronym SMARTER. This acronym helps describe optimal goals as:

- Specific: for example, "I want to become a better referee" is too vague and doesn't offer any direction whereas "I want to be ranked in the top five referees in my group" is much more specific.
- Measureable: optimal goals include clearly defined targets – for example, "I will read the rulebook for 20 minutes each day".
- Agreed: this describes the commitment aspect of optimal goals in which others who may have an influence are aware of the goal and record it.
- Realistic: optimal goals are characterised as challenging, yet achievable. This can be ensured by rating the difficulty of the goal from 1 (not at all difficult) to 10 (very difficult). Optimal goals rate somewhere between about 6 and 8 out of 10.
- Time-phased: each goal should have a clear target date.
- Evaluated: goals should be updated as the individual progresses to maintain optimal challenge and to set new goals once initial ones are realised.
- Rewards: incentives to reward successful achievement of goals are a key component of effective goal-setting.

Other goal setting tips:

- Write your goal in the first person.
- Identify the barriers that may get in your way to you achieving your goal, then develop a plan to overcome them.
- Use imagery to imagine yourself having achieved the goal.

Summary and conclusion

Mastering psychological skills will allow the official to develop the characteristics needed to cope with pressure performances. A commitment to critical self-analysis and reflection is the foundation upon which referees can build these skills. An open mind, a dedication to video/DVD review, consistent pre-event routines, ongoing use of imagery and role-playing and clear goals will all help the aspiring official progress through the performance levels and reach his or her performance potential.

Official's call (1)

Marika Humphreys-Baranova

I have found the chapter a very interesting read, especially when I contextualise the content against my experiences as an official and trainer of officials. Particularly reassuring was the realisation that the World Governing Body, the International Skating Union (ISU), appears to have a firm handle on good processes to train and facilitate functionality of officials at events. I will comment below on different sections and areas of the chapter.

Processes and demands of officiating

The ISU recruits former elite performers and high level coaches to their Technical Panels as they recognise that these individuals possess the characteristics highlighted in the chapter.

During Technical Panel training and examination, successful candidates demonstrate confidence, excellent communication skills, unshakable task focus, knowledge and real-time application of rules as well as the ability to recognise, review and correct mistakes.

The ISU guides its officials to strive for best practice by providing a thorough pre- and post-event routine for all of its officials including review of the code of ethics, review of officiating procedures, pre- and post-event meetings for review of officials' performance and independent third party review of event recordings. The use of all of these processes relates strongly to the later paragraphs of the chapter: Pre-event routines and Critical self-reflection through pre- and post-game briefings. I find that having a framework that is standard practice at all events calms and builds confidence in myself and my fellow officials.

Motivations to officiate

Of the Technical Panel officials that I have encountered, all endeavour to apply the rules with an even hand to give a consistent yardstick of achievement to the competing athletes. While every Championship level Technical Specialist is honoured by a high status appointment, it is the camaraderie and sense of using one's abilities for the benefit of the sport that is the main draw into this voluntary position.

Having been both coach to European and World Championship competitors and an Olympic level official, I have heard the locker room talk of both sides of the equation. While there are times when skaters/coaches may question or disagree with decisions made by the Technical Panel, every skater/coach is permitted to seek post-event feedback from the Technical Controller (administrative captain of the Technical Panel at each event) based on detailed notes of the Technical Panel. In my experience, this is a beneficial process allowing coaches and skaters to learn more about their performance and to develop strategy throughout the competitive season. It also goes some way to smoothing over any negative perceptions that athletes and coaches may hold about event officials.

However, if you were to take a survey in the stadium after an event, it would be easy to verify that there is a strong similarity in the patterns between the athlete/coach/fan/media versus officials' perceptions to which this chapter draws attention.

Psychological characteristics, commitment and quality practice

With regard to the core skills and characteristics mentioned in this chapter, it has been my assumption that the ISU recruits former elite athletes and coaches in order to capitalise on the tendency of these people to have already acquired many of these skills through their training/competition/work.

All officials in ice skating are part-time and volunteer their time. The fact that the ISU recruits primarily former elite skaters and coaches means that these officials have spent – and (preferably) continue to spend – significant time working on the ice every week. Whether coaching or performing, this is viewed as career and professional development (CPD) and an opportunity to keep the mind and eyes sharp, and to practise picking up visual cues with superior speed and accuracy in readiness for duties as an official. Technical Panel officials are also provided with footage from past events to practise observation and review processes.

Self-awareness/analysis and critical appraisal

This is another area where the ISU leads its officials by providing a framework of best practice. Technical Panels are encouraged to build a supportive team attitude at every event through discussion and review of the rules. Pre- and post-event meetings are mandatory and provide opportunities to communicate preferences for working practices, division of tasks and seeking methods for resolving contentious calls to maximise efficiency. This is extremely useful for us Technical Officials (TOs) as, at major championships and Olympic Games the event is televised, meaning we have 90 seconds or less to deliver an error-free evaluation of each performance.

Distraction/arousal control and clear and present tense focus

This is probably my favourite section of the chapter. The acid test for any Technical Panel is their efficiency when an unplanned event such as a fall or stumble occurs during an element (move or trick that needs to fulfil a set of criteria to achieve maximum point scoring potential). Division of work and the ability of each member of the Technical Panel to focus and prioritise analysis of the criteria fulfilled in order to arrive at the correct conclusion are essential. The process can become fraught and tense if just one Panel member loses their 'cool'.

The two stages for the Technical Panel are the real-time evaluation of each competitor's performance and an immediate post-performance review of any contentious calls. In stage 1 the competitors skate their routine while the Technical Panel identifies elements, evaluates and assigns levels of difficulty and identifies falls and illegal moves in real time. Stage 2 kicks in immediately after the skaters have finished their routine. The Technical Panel must review any contentious calls and use their detailed knowledge of the rules and variable speed replay to come to the right conclusion within the 90 second deadline.

The recommendation for stress exposure training to optimise performance of officials is excellent. Having been a trainer of Technical Specialists for the ISU for the past five years, I have employed a simplified version of this myself during the annual training course. As stressors, I have used scoring the performance of Technical Specialists on accuracy and speed to deliver the completed analysis, as well as observation by peers. The students report that initially they find this very stressful, but that over the week of preparation for the final examination they gain confidence and find they are able to prioritise and become more efficient at decision making. After reading this chapter I am now also planning to test the above real-time technique at this year's training seminar.

Overall, I found that I related well to this chapter. It describes processes we use, issues that we encounter, as well as techniques we can use in the future.

Official's call (2)

Chris White

My background and motivation

I was brought up in a rugby world. Cheltenham is a rugby town and I was born into it. My dad went to grammar school where they played and my brother played. I'd always taken an interest in the rules and laws – my dad was a teacher so that was in my blood. When I was eleven I wasn't picked for the school team so they made me touch judge (and the replacement at the same time). I loved the game, but it was different from the way kids love the game nowadays. The typical pathway for a young person now is to have an ambition to be a top referee. That wasn't really the case for me – I just liked it.

I've refereed a lot of small-sided school soccer – 200 to 300 games of school soccer as a teacher. I usually umpired the first 10–15 overs of my cricket matches if there was no umpire available. I still do it now. I'm a player-umpire, if you like. I have a similar mind-set that I'm going to do the job properly.

My teaching background has helped me in several ways. First of all it's about organising your environment, even before the game starts. "Right, this is what we're doing . . . right". A lot of people want to be organised. "We're gonna do this, then this and that's when I'll see you". It's not about telling people what you're going to do, it's just organising the environment. It's like teaching. There are 30 people who may or may not do what you want them to do and you have to find a way to make it work.

Passion and joy

Of the characteristics in this chapter, the ones that have been most beneficial to me in my development are passion and joy. There are so many times when you're sitting on the motorway on your own. There are so many things that can go wrong if you don't passionately love it. I watched this under 15s soccer game and the abuse they get – they must really love it.

"Man does seldom better than that which he does with passion". This rang a bell with me. The referees starting now, the ones who will survive the world pools of officiating are the ones who love what they are doing and the game. For example, I'm working with this young referee who officiated at a game last weekend, he did another game yesterday and wants to do another one this weekend.

Also, it's obvious to say the word 'commitment'. Everything revolves around your officiating if you're going to make it. The ones I see doing well, their refereeing is almost on a par with their family and work to the extent that you have to hold them back at times.

Finding solutions on the day

It's still the case that it's about finding a set of solutions that work for you on the day, in the sense that you don't know what the issues will be – you have to work out problems – you've got your perfect picture. It's like an electrician who asks what's broken and what are the clues as to why it's broken. What's in your toolbox to fix it? On a muddy day you may stand closer, say more at the breakdown and allow a little more leniency – so each game is different. Also, things are different at different levels – the junior and professional games are different.

Coping with on-field disruptions

Knowing you've missed something distracts me. Your head is suddenly full. For example, you have an advantage situation, then fast play, and a second event occurs – your head is now full – so your box can fill up very quickly and you have to slow it down. That might change with the more active television match official (TMO), but that extends the decision-making pathway. In the old days you had one look and made your decision; now you have one look, then you may have to look again and then, of course, you involve someone else in the process.

You have a good picture (it's that elite memory thing) and you replay what you've seen and you trust a mixture of instinct and judgement to which you apply the relevant law or protocol.

Above real-time training (ARTT)

A non-contact session is played ridiculously fast. It's the fastest 'live' practice you can do. Without defence it's flat out. It's flitting around all over the place. Other than using speeded video, the second way of ARTT is a professional contact session because it's full on. You're not looking at the wider context, the scoreline, the previous play or the position on the field; you're just looking at players smashing into each other every few seconds. The third way to do ARTT is a live scrum session where one scrum collapses, then they're straight back up again – it's back to back.

When I first started refereeing, rugby union was very limited on television so, if you sat in front of the television between 4pm and 5pm on Sunday, you'd probably miss the highlights with all the other people in the room. It was a wonderful distraction.

We've looked at flight simulator models and I've done a little to see if there's any crossover for the referee. The 'Ref cam' (now used on Sky's live rugby union broadcasts) will be a tool if we can harness it.

Performance feedback

I used to get – and our referees get – performance feedback in a few ways. First there is self-analysis of the game. Successful referees will recognise 90% of all aspects of that themselves. Then, for feedback, it's a mixture of official reviewers, mentors, referee coaches, etc. Players and coaches will tend to give you game-related things which shed light on what they're doing, which is the best thing I get from them – the technical stuff. We're doing our technical stuff and they're doing their technical stuff. They're changing all the time, so it's as well to know what's going on.

Self-belief and passion

You are always faced with "Was I right?" moments. And you have to be able to answer that – partly "Well, I was right before so I'm probably right now" – trust your instincts. It is your instincts – both gut and situational – that are probably right.

Pre-game routines

I always threw the ball against the wall of the changing room ten minutes before we started. The players would all look at me in the tunnel with disbelief. My answer to the player who asked "What are you doing?" was "I'd love to play today but I can't, I'm not good enough". It would fill a nervous moment – it would get hand/eye co-ordination going and everyone else laughed at me.

In big games I used to like to go outside and run around the in-goal area. I used to self-talk. It was unobtrusive, watching the teams warm up in a subconscious way. I used it before a game when I wanted to get myself in the right place. I wrote key notes before games – slightly different each time, but very basic: "Tackle – Tackler – Move"; just simple and key things to focus on.

Often the changing room was too full of administrators and non-performers so the pitch could be anywhere. I remember my first Tri-nations game and envisioning refereeing Northampton versus Leicester and thinking "It's no different here – it's just a game".

Training and self-talk

I was constantly thinking about refereeing; watching games and discussing matches and referee best practice in every sense: communicating, decision making, sharing experiences. I recognise it in other people. It's an obsession almost. Pretty sad. I still do it, but now I do it in the context of other referees.

When I first started, for the first ten years of refereeing I wasn't coached by anyone – no coach, no assessor. So I'd use "Dip – Bore – Bind – Legs", which was my self-talk for the scrum; simplistic, non-coached self-talk for the scrum. It helped me to recognise what was happening. They were the cues for me to look at. And the self-talk before the game in the 30 minutes before kick-off when on the pitch. And the third time is post-match or before the next match in difficult fitness training – often 'downloading' frustrations or angers or conversations – people who'd got to me and I'd feel I'd work it through while under physical pressure. It was a sort of catharsis. There'd be a massive amount of vision going on in my head. There'd be a lot of self-talk going on when I was interval training because you wanted to get there. Downloading frustrations and finding solutions in your head. I learned that I had to find a solution in my head. You're always looking to turn the negatives into positives.

Imagery

I used to use imagery. Pictures of the perfect scrum and the perfect contest (the tackle). I had a very strong picture of what was right for the game. I used this in preparation for the game. During the game I think imagery is constant and post-game you're constantly taking pictures. I used mental rehearsal to plan my delivery to players and also to replay it afterwards.

Goal-setting

I used goal-setting. This is definitely a standard part of refereeing nowadays as it's a big part of our lives. There's a performance part of refereeing, so there are goals there all the time. I would record the games down retrospectively. I didn't write down my goals as I thought one game and one decision at a time.

Refereeing the World Cup semi-final: it caught me by surprise to be in contention. I recognise how it happened as you go through the rounds. But it's not like playing. You can win your way to a Wimbledon final but you can't win your way to refereeing the final. For example, if England are playing, I can't referee it. If your style isn't the right style, if a team plays badly and you get drawn into that. You may referee better but it's a lot harder if the scrums collapse all game and sometimes that's not your choice. Referee selection is about perception whereas, for an athlete, if you win a game you're through regardless of whether you're the best.

Probably the biggest psychological problems for me were travel, time away and protecting your performance. The onfield bit – I used to feel alive on the pitch. I just used to love being out there. The bit on the pitch I just loved it. I just really enjoyed refereeing. I just get so much pleasure from it.

Nowadays there's less foul play and you get help with foul play. The game 'kicking off' used to be a real challenge. It was yours to deal with. You had to referee. I red-carded 75 players in 32 years, and 45 were in the first 10 years.

Summary

Overall, there's some good stuff in the chapter and the book. I think this will resonate with a lot of people who care about officiating or if you are a coach or a referee or someone interested in the madness of officiating. I enjoyed reading it. There are also practical things. For example, I'm going to use the page on goal-setting with my Scholarship students!

References

[1] Wolfson, S., & Neave, N. (2007). Coping under pressure: Cognitive strategies for maintaining confidence among soccer referees. *Journal of Sport Behavior, 30*, 232–47.

[2] Simmons, P. (2006). Tackling abuse of officials: Attitudes and communication skills of experienced football referees. Paper presented to the Australia and New Zealand Communication Association Conference, University of Adelaide, Adelaide, Australia.

[3] Balch, M. J., & Scott, D. (2007). Contrary to popular belief, refs are people too! Personality and perceptions of officials. *Journal of Sport Behavior, 30*, 3–20.

[4] Philippe, F. L., Vallerand, R. J., Andrianarisoa, J., & Brunel, P. (2009). Passion in referees: Examining their affective and cognitive experiences in sport situations. *Journal of Sport and Exercise Psychology, 31*, 77–96.

[5] McCaffrey, N. & Orlick, T. (1989). Mental factors related to excellence among top professional golfers. *International Journal of Sport Psychology, 20*, 256–78.

[6] Orlick, T., & Partington, J. (1988). Mental links to excellence. *The Sport Psychologist, 2*, 105–30.

[7] Greenleaf, C. A., Gould, D., & Dieffenbach, K. (2001). Factors influencing Olympic performance: Interviews with Atlanta and Nagano U.S. Olympians. *Journal of Applied Sport Psychology, 13*, 179–209.

[8] Gould, D., Dieffenbach, K., & Moffett, A. (2002). Psychological characteristics and their development in Olympic champions. *Journal of Applied Sport Psychology, 14*, 172–204.

[9] Abbott, A., Collins, D., & Sowerby, K. (2007). Developing the potential of young people in sport. SportScotland, Edinburgh.

[10] MacNamara, A. (2011). Psychological characteristics of developing excellence. In D. Collins, H. Richards, & C. Button (Eds). *Performance psychology – Developing a peak performance culture* (pp. 47–64). Elsevier.

[11] Jones, G., Hanton, S., & Connaughton, D. (2002). What is this thing called mental toughness? An investigation of elite sport performers. *Journal of Applied Sport Psychology*, *14*, 205–18.

[12] Eysenck, M.W., Derakshan, N., Santos, R. (2007). Anxiety and cognitive performance: Attentional control theory. *Emotion*, *7*, 336–53.

[13] Driskell, J.E., & Johnson, J. H. (1998). Stress exposure training. In J. A. Cannon-Bowers, & E. Salas (Eds). *Making decisions under stress: Implications for individual and team training* (pp. 191–217). Washington, DC: American Psychological Association.

[14] Lorains, M., MacMahon, C., Ball, K., & Mahoney, J. (2011). Above real time training for team invasion sport skills. *International Journal of Sports Science and Coaching*, *6*, 537–44.

[15] Lorains, M., Ball, K., & MacMahon, C. (2013). An above real time training intervention for sport decision making. *Psychology of Sports and Exercise*, *14*, 670–4.

[16] Lorains, M., Ball, K., & MacMahon, C. (2013). Expertise differences in a video decision-making task: Speed influences on performance. *Psychology of Sports and Exercise*, *14*, 293–7.

[17] Bandura, A. (1977). Self-efficacy: Toward a unifying theory of behavioral change. *Psychological Review*, *84*, 191–215.

[18] Bandura, A. (1997). *Self-efficacy: The exercise of control*. New York: Freeman and Co.

[19] Guillén, F., & Feltz, D. (2011). A conceptual model of referee efficacy. *Frontiers in Psychology*, *2*(25).

[20] Mascarenhas, D. R. D., Collins, D., & Mortimer, P. (2005). Elite refereeing performance: Developing a model for sport science support. *The Sport Psychologist*, *19*, 364–79.

[21] Helsen, W. F., Hodges, N. J., Van Winckel, J., & Starkes, J. L. (2000). The roles of talent, physical precocity and practice in the development of soccer expertise. *Journal of Sport Sciences*, *18*, 727–36.

[22] Helsen, W. F., Starkes, J. L., & Hodges, N. J. (1998). Team sports and the theory of deliberate practice. *Journal of Sport and Exercise Psychology*, *20*, 12–34.

[23] Australian Institute of Sport (2008). *Concentration: Strategies for improving concentration*. http://www.ausport.gov.au/ais/sssm/psychology/brainwaves/factsheets/concentration (accessed 14 February 2014).

[24] Cautella, J. R., & Wisocki, P. A. (1977). The thought stopping procedure: Description, application, and learning theory interpretations. *The Psychological Record*, *2*, 255–64.

[25] Rothkopf, E. & Billington, M. (1979). Goal-guided learning from text: Inferring a descriptive processing model from inspection times and eye movements. *Journal of Educational Psychology*, *71*, 310–27.

[26] Bandura, A., & Cervone, D. (1983). Self-evaluative and self-efficacy mechanisms governing the motivational effects of goal systems. *Journal of Personality and Social Psychology*, *45*, 1017–28.

[27] Locke, E. (1968). Toward a theory of task motivation and incentives. *Organizational Behavior and Human Performance*, *3*, 157–89.

[28] Baddeley, A. D. (2001). Is working memory still working? *American Psychologist*, *56*, 851.

[29] Collins, D. J. (1998). In the event. (How) Does anxiety affect performance? Invited keynote presentation, British Psychological Society Annual Conference, Brighton, April.

8

TECHNOLOGY

Introduction

In the Euro 2012 soccer match between England and Ukraine, a shot by Ukraine's striker Marko Devic´ was cleared from just behind the goal line by England's defender John Terry. This was clearly visible to all television viewers. Unfortunately, none of the referees perceived the ball to have passed the line and, consequently, no goal was awarded to the Ukrainian team that finally lost the game 0–1 and was eliminated from the tournament. Inevitably, this incident reopened a debate about technological aids for referee decisions in soccer. Soccer associations are frequently blamed for leaving referees unnecessarily uninformed because they don't allow them to use helpful technologies, such as video replay, in critical situations. Although there have been some recent changes to this rigid attitude, such as FIFA recently allowing goal-line technologies,[1] knowing about these regulations, one can get the impression that technical support is rather uncommon in sports officiating. In contrast to this impression, there is actually a long history of technology-based assessments of sport performance and even video review is now common in many sports.

In this chapter we will present an overview of the most common technical aids that are used by sports officials. We will also discuss the pros and cons of technological aids as well as their reliability and validity. Unfortunately, this must be done mainly on the basis of individual cases because systematic scientific research on this topic is rather rare to date.

As an interesting side aspect, we also report constraints that some sports put on the frequency of technology-based decisions. Finally, we will take a look at the possibilities that modern technologies offer for the training of officials.

Assessment and validation of sports performance

Timing

In many sports the measurement of time plays an important role. This is most obvious in races like the 100 metres in track and field. Here the accurate assessment of each athlete's performance serves not only as a way to establish the correct ranking within a race but also for comparisons between races or even for historical comparisons (records). For a long time hand-held stopwatches did a good job for this, but even the most accurate ones depend on human judgement and reactions. Therefore, electronic timing systems have replaced hand-held watches for most purposes. In principle, the systems used in sports today can be accurate to less than 0.001 of a second (for an interesting exception see Box 8.1). Nevertheless, very close races are also decided on the basis of photo-finish video cameras. These cameras can scan a thin line aligned with the finish line up to 3000 times per second. At best they can be used as a kind of backup system in order to confirm a difference between two or more close competitors. For example, at the Olympic Games in Beijing in 2008, the 100 meter butterfly race was very close; Michael Phelps (USA) won by only one-hundredth of a second ahead of Milorad Cavic (Serbia) on his way to a historic gain of eight gold medals. It seemed obvious that Michael Phelps had stopped the chronograph first, but the recorded video images were not so clear about this result.

BOX 8.1 THE TIMING MECHANISM

The sport of fencing received unusual attention during the London Olympics 2012 but did not make good use of this platform. It was the last second of the semi-final of the women's epee between German Britta Heidemann and Shin Lam from South Korea that provoked a major controversy. In a thrilling bout no winner was found and, with the score at 5–5, it was to be decided in 'sudden death'. Shin had been given priority – that is, the onus to score within the next minute was on Heidemann – whereas a draw would have been enough for the South Korean to proceed to the final and fight for the gold medal. After three double hits in the last second of sudden death, giving no contestant a point, Shin thought she had made it. However, the automatic timing mechanism did not signal the end of the sudden death minute. The Austrian referee, Barbara Csar, decided in agreement with both contestants to reset the clock once more from zero to one second, giving Heidemann a fourth chance to attack within a single second. This time she did score a hit and was declared the winner. Shin broke down in tears on the piste and her coach immediately launched an appeal against the referee's decision to reset the clock. It took the officials almost half an hour to reject the appeal and confirm Heidemann's victory. The German celebrated while the stadium announcer tried to explain to the audience, which by now had completely taken the side of the sobbing South Korean, why she

(continued)

(continued)

still remained on the piste. According to the rules, her leaving would void her coach's second appeal automatically. The desperate fencer crying on the piste has become one of the iconic images of the London Olympics, and this semi-final raised the question why a highly technologised sport such as fencing – which employs video evidence, electronic devices and scoring lights to indicate a hit – still relies on a timing mechanism that measures time in whole seconds only and not in centiseconds. The referee was later heavily criticised by commentators and spectators, and Korean bloggers even published her home address on the internet since they believe Lam was cheated out of her chance for the gold medal. Officials of the International Fencing Federation later confirmed the correctness of Csar's factual decision but still offered the South Korean a consolation prize to recognise her sportsmanship.

Strangely, and largely unnoticed, in 2009 the official timekeeper in Beijing, the Swiss company OMEGA, admitted that Milorad Cavic touched the wall first, although not as forcefully as Michael Phelps. Thus, even the most accurate time keeping systems can only be as good as the devices with which they are started and stopped (if not automatically). If this holds true for such a well-understood technical problem as timing, it is of even bigger concern with the increasingly popular video review.

Video review

In contrast to soccer, video review has been established in many sports in order to assist officials with difficult decisions. For example, Television Match Official (TMO) decision analysis was introduced in rugby union in 1999. It provides an opportunity for the referee to check any try decisions that are doubtful or difficult and, more recently, has been extended to include incidents of foul play. Obviously, this opportunity has met with wide acceptance from referees, players, coaches, supporters and the press. A report from 2002 states that an additional benefit has been the reduction of controversial decisions made by referees that may have had a material impact on the outcome of a game.[2] This general positive appraisal of video review is shared by officials from most sports where it is used. However, here we like to point to the fact that most of the research that we discussed in Chapter 5 about biases in officials' decision making was conducted with video materials. Consequently, there is no reason to assume that officials using video review in competitions are immune to these biases. Just because decisions become more accepted does not mean that they are more accurate. In addition, the mode of video replay (e.g., slow motion) can change the entire way a body movement is viewed, processed and judged.[3] Again, the question arises as to the standard of comparison. If video-based decisions are evaluated on the basis of video analyses, the consistency is inevitably high. Thus, we need more independent studies on the validity of video-based decisions in order to determine their benefit in this regard. The following two examples will highlight some additional problems that can come up with video review.

In the London 2012 Olympics men's team gymnastics final, Kōhei Uchimura from Japan fell from the pommel horse during his dismount. The judges recognised the lack of a dismount and lowered the difficulty value of his routine accordingly. The Japanese coaches appealed the scoring on this performance as Uchimura still landed on his feet and they felt this should have counted as a full dismount, albeit with serious deductions. Before the protest, Great Britain was positioned to get silver behind China and the Ukraine to finish with a bronze. The protest by the Japanese team led to a longer video review by the competition judges. Even with the help of video review, it seemed to be very difficult to reach a decision. Fifteen minutes after the end of the competition, Uchimura's routine score was revised upwards by 0.7 points and the team promoted back to second place. It was the first time that a video review-based correction had a direct impact on an Olympic medal decision.

In golf, TV evidence was used to determine whether a ball at rest had moved. Even a TV viewer could initiate this review process. For example, in the BMW Championship in September 2013, Tiger Woods tried to remove a twig from beside his ball before playing his third shot on the first hole. He felt his ball had only oscillated before he ran up a double-bogey six, but high-definition video footage showed that it had slightly shifted its position and his score was amended to a quadruple-bogey eight. Of course, Tiger Woods is subjected to more television coverage than any other player so he has a higher chance of being penalised on the basis of TV evidence than others. In fact, the rules have been changed since this incident and now it has been decided that a player is not penalised in circumstances where the fact that the ball has changed location could not reasonably have been seen without the use of enhanced technology.

These two examples from gymnastics and golf point to important questions that officials have to deal with when allowing video review under certain circumstances. What happens when the video material provides no conclusive answer to the question asked? And how are we to deal with situations when only limited or even no video material is available (e.g., due to technical problems or because cameras were just angled in another direction)? This last question also points to a frequent argument against advanced technologies: they often involve extra costs and are only available at an elite level. Thus, decision rules are different on elite levels than on sub-elite levels and officials have to adapt depending on the level of their assignment. Moreover, it is an open question if the gains of a video review system really justify the extra costs from an economic perspective. For example, the economist Vani K. Borooah from the University of Ulster suggests that the money that is invested in cricket's decision review system would be better invested directly in umpires.[4] He found that the review system helped to increase the percentage of correct decisions in cricket from 93.1 per cent to 95.8 per cent, but at the cost of about US$100,000 per match. Imagine what could be done with this money in the education and training of umpires (see Chapter 9).

In all of the examples so far, video review was used to provide additional information to officials in order to support their decision making. However, more and more development is going on that aims to replace the official by technical systems. For example, colleagues from Pakistan developed a system for the automatic analysis of video data in cricket.[5] Here the fielding team can dismiss a batsman from scoring through a run-out, i.e., the batsman fails to enter an area before three stumps are dislodged in that area. Normally, an extra umpire makes the 'run-out/not-out' decision through video technology. With the novel technology called A-Eye that makes this decision autonomously, this umpire could be replaced. In principle, one of the most advanced technologies in this field, Hawk-Eye,[6] shares this goal. We will describe this technology and situation in more detail below.

Hawk-Eye

The Hawk-Eye system was developed by the British mathematician Paul Hawkins in 2001. Nowadays it is used – among other sports – in tennis, cricket and snooker, with a system for soccer being developed. In this system, several cameras are set up around the playing area. They are carefully calibrated so that a three-dimensional position of the ball can be established. The trajectory of the ball is monitored during the entire duration of play. In cricket, the system is used to judge leg before wicket calls, as it can predict what the path of the ball would have been if it had not been interrupted by the batsman. In tennis it has been used since 2006 to indicate whether the ball bounced in or not. Questions have been raised about the accuracy of Hawk-Eye, despite claims from the manufacturer. As with any such system, it is unlikely to be correct 100 per cent of the time; there is still measurement error, even if low. For example, in tennis it is indicated that the mean error in the position of the tennis ball is 3.6 millimetres. However, no information is available about the distribution and dispersion of errors or the conditions under which errors are greater or smaller. In response to this, some colleagues argue that the public understanding of measurement errors and confidence intervals could be enhanced if decision aids such as the Hawk-Eye system were to present their results in a different way.[7] They think that there is a danger that Hawk-Eye, as it is currently used, could inadvertently cause naïve viewers to overestimate the ability of technological devices to resolve disagreement among humans because measurement errors are not made salient. For example, virtual reconstructions can easily be taken by viewers to show 'exactly what really happened'. As an alternative, they suggest that confidence levels might be measured and represented in a readily comprehensible manner. They argue that decision aids could add to the enjoyment of sport and to a better public understanding of the limits and possibilities of technologies if their capabilities were presented in such a transparent way.

Of course, technologies like Hawk-Eye can also be used beyond certain in/out decisions for the general study of officials' (and players') decision accuracy.

For example, George Mather analysed the records of 1,473 challenges made by 246 professional tennis players (or doubles teams) during ATP tennis tournaments worldwide during 2006 and 2007.[8] Among other results, he found that line judges (as well as players) are remarkably accurate at judging ball bounce position, with a positional uncertainty of less than 40 millimetres. However, line judges are more reliable than players. He also found that judgements are more difficult for balls bouncing near the base and service lines than those bouncing near the side and central lines. This is a good example of the multitude of interesting information that modern technologies can provide the official beyond their main function as decision aids.

Rules of technology-based decisions

With all the novel technologies available that can either assist or even replace an official's decision, the question arises: under which circumstances should they be used? Always? Every time an official wants to use them? Or only if somebody protests against a decision? Different sports answer this question in different ways:

- In tennis, Hawk-Eye can be used only if one of the players challenges a line call. The challenge can refer either to the player's or his or her opponent's shot. For this, each player receives two challenges per set. The challenged situation will immediately be checked by the Hawk-Eye system and displayed on a video screen. Officials are then bound to accept the Hawk-Eye ruling. If it turns out that the player is correct with a challenge, then he or she retains the same number of challenges. Effectively, players have an unlimited number of correct challenges to make. However, if the player is incorrect with a challenge, then one of the challenges is lost. Additional rules state that each player will receive an additional challenge during a tie-break and that challenges may not be carried over from one set to another.
- In gymnastics, video review can only be used by an independent and neutral panel of officials (i.e., composed of persons who were not involved in the original scoring). It requires the inquiry of a gymnast's coach that must be made immediately after the publication of the score and shall concern only the difficulty score of a routine (in contrast to the execution score). The panel will compare the original score with the video review and make a final decision on the difficulty score. It is not allowed to complain against the score of an opponent. At European Championships, the inquiry requires an agreement of payment of 300 Euros for the first complaint, 500 Euros for the second complaint and 1000 Euros for the third and any further complaints. If the inquiry is accepted, this sum will be reimbursed.
- In field hockey, a video umpire has the opportunity to use replays from any camera angle as necessary before reaching a decision about goal situations. However, this requires a referral by the match umpire. The match umpire

can make a referral every time he or she feels insecure in deciding whether or not a goal has been legally scored. On the basis of the video review, the video umpire provides a recommendation, e.g., 'goal', which can be used by the match umpire for the final decision. In addition, each team is allowed one team referral request during any match. It is restricted to decisions within the 23 metre areas relating to the award (or non-award) of goals, penalty strokes and penalty corners. If the video umpire finds no clear reason to change the match umpire's original decision, the referring team loses its right of referral. Otherwise the team retains its right of referral.

In all of these sports, technology use is limited in order to save time. In addition, it is obvious that some of these rules try to restrict the use of technologies to certain situations where athletes or coaches are quite confident that the decision by an official is wrong. The (implicit) assumption of the rule makers seems to be that, otherwise, athletes and coaches would complain about any decision that is not to their advantage. Indeed, a recent study on over 2,000 challenges by tennis players in 35 tournaments suggests that their decisions of whether to challenge umpires' calls are not only driven by their corresponding perceptions but also by their motivation.[9] For example, they are more likely to challenge when the stakes are higher (e.g., in the final set).

Assistants in communication

In all sports, technical assistants have been introduced at least on an elite level in order to support the communication between officials or with athletes, players and spectators. For example, every modern stadium or sports hall has a big video screen that can be used to display officials' decisions in detail. This seems to be a matter of course and almost natural. Sometimes large screen display is even a necessary part of performance measurement (e.g., start signals) and is closely integrated in the measurement technology (see the section on Timing above). The same holds for technical systems that support the general organisation and management of a competition (e.g., in gymnastics).

There has only been a small amount of research to date on whether and how these assistants change officials' behaviour and if they are, indeed, all for the best of the official. For example, older research on so-called conformity processes already shows that gymnastics judges can be influenced by the scores of other judges that are displayed on a television screen during a competition.[10] Sometimes associations leave it to the officials to decide if they will use the technologies that are offered. For example, in soccer some referee teams use wireless headsets that facilitate communication over longer distances whereas, for others, this seems not to be necessary.

In general, we suggest that officials carefully compare the advantages and disadvantages of each new communication technology that is offered to them before they are introduced as an inherent part of their officiating.

The acceptance of technologies

In a pragmatic manner, one can argue that any technology for officials fulfils its purpose if officials are more confident with it and the acceptance of their decisions increases. In fact, a few studies suggest that this is indeed the case. For example, the already cited report on TMOs in rugby found that the decision of the TMO is generally accepted by the spectator, supporter and press as being accurate and thus removes pressure from the on-field official.[2] The reported statistics also indicate that the on-field referee has adapted well to the involvement of the TMO by only using the TMO on average once per game, with a 91 per cent accuracy being achieved.

In two studies the Australian Rene Leveux interviewed officials from various sports including taekwondo, cricket, soccer, rugby league, rugby union and tennis about their experiences with technical decision aids.[11, 12] He found that, when used, the technology does provide a mechanism to facilitate ensuring the correctness of the decision. The success of the introduction of the decision support technology is dependent on its usability, appropriate application and acceptance by the officials and the participants of the match. Through the diligent use and application of appropriate technologies, they can be used as an effective aid to refereeing. For example, illegal tactics and play were commonplace prior to the introduction of the use of technology to assist the referee. These areas, however, have been dramatically reduced and, to a certain extent, eliminated. Consequently, these introduced technologies have been a major contributor to the provision of a fairer platform for competition and have led to improved player performance. Especially in taekwondo, it was found that the diligent use and application of technologies provided mechanisms to greatly improve the correctness of decisions by being an effective aid to the referee's decision-making process, which contributed to the success of the event. In addition, the implementation and use of these technologies is considered to provide a more attractive competition.

Together, the available studies so far strongly support the introduction of technical aids for sports officials. While technical aids were cautiously and very sceptically received by refereeing officials initially, they are now accepted at the elite level and have provided an innovative and effective support mechanism to provide the platform for both increased transparency and correctness of officials' decision making in the game. However, we also note that, in these studies, nothing has been asked about the costs that come with the introduction of new technologies.

Officials' training

Surely most technologies that we have discussed so far can also serve officials as tools in their education and training. For example, we have already provided an example of using the Hawk-Eye system to gain information about the accuracy of linesmen in tennis.[8] Many such systems provide data that include specific feedback about the performance of officials and, thus, hints on how to improve their training.

In addition, various technologies like video simulations and online training tools have been developed specifically to support their decision-making training (see Chapter 9). Furthermore, every technology that can help athletes to improve their performance can also be helpful for officials. For example, head-mounted cameras have become frequent (and cheap) and can be easily used to receive feedback about one's own behaviour on the pitch in training (and competition).[13] Together, we think that officials should be open-minded towards the multitude of possibilities that modern technologies offer for education and training.

Summary and conclusion

Officials usually need to combine several pieces of information for a decision. Due to the difficulty of this task, it will never be possible to achieve 100 per cent correct decisions. Some incidents are so hard to decide upon that, even with repeated viewings of the video recording, many referees cannot agree on a decision.[14] It is important to emphasise that this is not because of the officials' skills. Some situations in the course of a sports competition are just so ambiguous that an objectively correct decision simply cannot be determined.

Referring to the example we used at the start of this chapter, what about the meaningfulness of technical aids such as a goal camera and video review in foul situations? From a psychological perspective, this question must be answered clearly: video evidence makes sense only in situations where the correct decision is objectively ascertainable. Whether or not the ball has crossed the goal line could be such a situation; if a camera is positioned optimally, it can very quickly and clearly indicate whether the ball was in the goal or not. However, technical systems such as Hawk-Eye are also not 100 per cent accurate. In the millimeter range there remains a certain measurement uncertainty. Overall, a goal camera appears to make sense, especially since the (low) probability of error in technical systems is apparently more acceptable than in humans.

Once again, it looks quite differently for video review of situations like foul play in soccer. In many controversial foul situations it cannot be clearly ascertained whether the incident is a foul or not. Thus, in these situations it is impossible to get to an objectively correct decision. The problem would just be passed on to the next instance – the 'bogeyman' would no longer be the referee on the pitch but the video referee. While the video referee may well be better able than the referee on the pitch to determine the correct decision in some situations, this is not valid for all situations, as is frequently suggested by proponents of video review. In addition, the video review of foul play would entail considerable costs. An obvious disadvantage would also be that the authority of the referee on the pitch would be weakened. Just this authority, however, is crucial for his or her successful management of a game (see Chapter 6). In soccer, it is also unclear how to deal with the events that happen between the referee's decision and a possible correction by the video referees off the pitch. In addition, a complex set of rules must be developed to guide how and under what circumstances video review is involved in the decision process. As we have seen, sports where hitherto video information can be consulted for certain decisions (e.g., rugby, field hockey, tennis, gymnastics) deal very differently with this problem, and it is an open question as to which of these models is most suitable for soccer matches. Finally, most users of computers know that sometimes even (or especially) the best technical systems may develop a tendency to fail in important moments. What then?

Technical aids can be useful assistants for officials, but their value depends strongly on how they are used. And one tool will never replace the personality of an official and their communication and social skills that are necessary to turn a competition into a great event.

Official's call (1)

Holger Albrecht

Introduction

By and large, this chapter covers all the technical tools that are of significance for men's artistic gymnastics judges, at least in international competitions like the FIG World Championships. It starts with the verification of the maximum duration of a floor exercise by a timer and leads to video control for the determination of a routine's difficulty score, which was introduced in 2005. I think that the rules of technology-based decisions are closely linked to each of these technologies and, thus, could also be treated directly within the first subheading.

Assessment and validation of sports performance

At first, during a gymnastics competition, several time standards need to be monitored concerning, for example, the warm-up period of a gymnast or the 30 seconds after the start signal in which he is expected to begin his exercise. Of course, these periods need not be measured in milliseconds and, in principle, a normal stopwatch could fulfil this purpose. At international competitions the corresponding timing devices are embedded in the general steering programme of the competition and normally they work without problems. However, sometimes a delay of time measurement occurs after a gymnast has fallen from an apparatus. He has the right to rest or recuperate for up to 30 seconds before he continues his exercise. Because falls are typically unexpected, the head judge sometimes needs a moment of reflection before he starts and announces the timing. Thus, some gymnasts may be awarded more time for recovery than others. This potential source of inequity could be avoided with an automatic timing device that starts the moment the athlete hits the ground.

In gymnastics, the final score of an exercise is established by the addition of the scores for difficulty and execution. The difficulty score is determined by a routine's value parts (and their combinations) and the execution score refers to the evaluation of faults. Concerning the assessment of the difficulty score, video control was implemented in 2005. The FIG provided IRCOS (Instant Replay and Information System), which allows a quick check for the difficulty to resolve possible ambiguity. Given that the rules for the evaluation of value parts are really complicated in parts and sometimes depend on small movements (e.g., touching or not touching a pommel on the pommel horse), it can sometimes happen that even the most experienced judges are unsure about what they have seen. With the help of this system, most of these cases can be clarified within an instant. Thus, I find this system really helpful in order to award the correct difficulty score. The case described in the chapter concerning the team competition at the Olympic Games in London 2012 where it took about 15 minutes before the final score (and ranking) was announced was one of the extremely rare cases when even the video control provided no clear answer.

So far, video analysis has been used in competitions only for the assessment of the difficulty score and not for the execution score. Currently, there are some tests of the video-based measurement of the duration of hold elements. In general, hold elements like the cross on rings need to be held for two seconds for full recognition. It would be a great help for the execution judges if this duration could be reliably assessed in future competitions.

Rules of technology-based decisions

When the video control was introduced in 2005 it could be used in any case of ambiguity. Unfortunately, the rules were changed in 2009 and now it can only be used if an inquiry for a difficulty score has been launched. It must be made by a gymnast's coach immediately after the publication of his score or, at the very latest, before the end of the exercise of the following gymnast. It requires an agreement of payment of about 300 Euros for the first inquiry and even more for additional inquiries. If the inquiry is accepted, this sum is reimbursed. The potential costs help to prevent pure tactical inquiries. However, in my opinion, video control should be accessible to difficulty judges at any time they are unsure about the correct score. The current procedure creates a tendency to judge in favour of the gymnast if there are doubts. This could be a disadvantage for gymnasts who present a perfect performance that leaves no doubts.

Assistants in communication

At international competitions, all judges type their score directly into a system that automatically calculates the final score and uses this information for the publication of results, rankings, etc. So far, I have never experienced problems with these systems and find them extremely helpful in order to support the judges in focusing on their main task – determining the correct score.

Due to the seating arrangement that is prescribed by the Code of Points, there can often be quite some distance between judges at an apparatus. In order to resolve controversies directly and quickly, a good old-fashioned telephone connection has proved to be very helpful.

Officials' training

There are a multitude of video-based tools available for gymnastics judges for training as well as for the evaluation of judges' performances at competitions. For example, these tools are provided directly as a kind of by-product by IRCOS. In general, I agree that they are of great value and we are lucky that nowadays we have so many technical possibilities that are easily accessible. I also welcome the scientific development of additional tools that aim to help practice the specific judgement task in order to suppress sources of potential biases. However, in my opinion, the best training for a gymnastics judge is still to go to the gym and observe gymnasts during their training. The direct contact with them and their striving to fulfil the demands of the Code de Points will create much better access to the real difficulties that matter in judging gymnastics.

Official's call (2)

Graham Hughes

How important is technology in rugby union officiating?

Technology in rugby union is another tool in the referee's bag. Video technology is used for referrals where there may be 'material incidents' which may affect the game scoreline and for incidents of foul play. So, the TMO can be called upon for any decision relating to an in-goal (try) decision. *Material incidents* are those which may directly impact upon the scoreline. If video replay were used the same way in soccer for example, it would be where you have a questionable offside decision. If the player then shot the ball over the bar, it would not be used. If the offside decision led to the player scoring, then the review would be used to see if there was a 'clear and obvious' offside. In rugby union the on-field referee will begin by asking one of three questions:

1. Is it a try – yes or no?
2. Can you give me a reason why I cannot award a try?
3. But for the act of foul play – probable try or no try?

We work quite closely with the TV producer, so it's very important he or she is very clear on what we want to see, to ensure that the process is swift. The producers are pretty good at understanding the game so will often know what to look for, but the RFU has now introduced a clearer protocol to make it easier for the videotape operators (who are often not as rugby savvy as the producers) and hence quicker for the audience. The on-field referee will also ask – who, what, when and where? So, for example, the referee might say, "Try – yes or no? Can you check the actions of number 5 green at the last ruck about 10 seconds ago on the defensive 22 metre line?" This has made it easier for the videotape operators and, as a consequence, the process is quicker.

So, for example, in a recent Six Nations game between Wales and France, Sam Warburton, the Welsh openside flanker, was tackled and reached forward to the line to place the ball down. I was called upon to review the ball placement. The producer reported to me (within about 10–15 seconds) that he had four angles. The first three were at ground level so it was hard to see whether the ball had crossed the line, but I was able to consider if it was controlled and if he was still in possession. The final angle, which was further away but high, showed that it was over the line so I was able to report that there was no problem with the grounding. The referee Alain Roland then asked if I could check for a knock-on in the previous ruck. I was able to confirm that this was okay after seeing two angles and the try was awarded. The process did take some time, but we got the right decision. Previously we've had problems with the production team wanting to show every plausible angle (televised games will have at least twelve cameras at every game nowadays) and wanting us to wait until the on-field referee was in shot before reporting back to them, but this has improved.

If I see definite foul play as the TMO I can report it live to the referee. If it's just potential foul play, I would talk to him at the next stoppage and the referee can watch the screen in the stadium and will make a decision – if he can – based on the screen, so the stadium screen can also be used.

In 2012/2013 the RFU trialled using the TMO for incidents of foul play in addition to in-goal decisions. As a consequence of this trial and another in South Africa, the IRB decided that they would stick to reviewing only up to two phases prior to a scoring play. When this extension came in there were concerns that it was going to slow the game down but, interestingly, that seems to have been accepted because they can see that it isn't actually taking that long and we're getting more decisions right. Typically, we have about two or three TMO referrals during a game. You can usually see when it's coming so you're ready for it – though there was a case of a TMO having to quit because every time the referee made the TV signal to refer a decision he was having panic attacks.

One of the biggest impacts that technology has had upon officiating is simply in the timekeeping because it is now done so openly. It appears on the screens, at the grounds – everybody is aware of how long is left, so it reduces the controversy. In the Six Nations the TMOs keep time and in the Premiership there are designated timekeepers where it is linked to the on-screen time on the game clock on the TV broadcast pictures. The on-field referee is still the judge of time, but the mechanics of it is now open.

We also use an open microphone system. This allows people at the ground and on TV to hear the communication between the team of five officials (referee, two assistants, fourth official on the sideline and the TMO). The referee's microphone is open whereas all the others are push-to-talk to avoid cross-chatter. This really helps with clarity so that everyone can hear why certain decisions are made.

Technology is an area where we can learn from other sports. We've always looked at rugby league in terms of how they use the TMO. That's partly how we come up with the protocols. They have a lot more flexibility in their system, whereas in rugby union we feel that the technology is there to support rather than interfere.

Who knows what forms of technology will be embraced in the future. I think the balance is about right at the moment. I'm not sure I agree with the idea of captain's challenge as they have in rugby league, which is similar to the systems used in cricket and tennis where players can contest an official's decision. In 2013/2014 the TMO system is still under global trial. Some unions want to eliminate forward pass decisions from referral, but I think that it could create more controversy when a 'clear and obvious' forward pass has been made that the TMO cannot adjudicate on.

Currently, referees are using GPS technologies to analyse their physical performance to inform their training programmes, but I'm not sure how that might benefit the consumer. Some production companies are experimenting with a camera on a pole that they use for lineouts for the viewing side of things, which they think gives a better view, but I'm not sure how that would benefit the officials. Also, a kicking camera has been used that is placed directly behind the kicker when taking a penalty kick. This gives a good perspective to see if the kick is on target, and it has even been used by placing it in front of the ball. Apparently it didn't interfere with the kicker's strike, but the reality is I'm not sure how a two-dimensional image would be better than the two three-dimensional images that the assistants provide from their position directly under the posts. It would be a brave man who over-rules their perspective with something provided by a video camera.

Some sports are perhaps a bit wary of introducing technology in their sports but I think they need to take a leap of faith and trial these things. There were a lot of critics in rugby union when we began to use TMOs, with people seeing it as a threat or challenging the values of honesty in our sport, but it seems pretty accepted now. Actually, making the referee's communication public in rugby union seems to have enhanced the appreciation for the referee. The feeling is often that it will change the game forever, but the reality is the game is forever changing. Being able to embrace technology to support the referee is a good thing.

TMO training

The Premiership referees meet about every two weeks and always includes a TMO. There are a number of things on the agenda, but there is always a review of decisions. In addition, the TMOs meet three times a year. At that meeting we will review probably about 14 clips – these will be a selection of 'controversial' decisions that the TMOs self-select in order to generate discussion. We don't necessarily all agree at first, but the idea is that we discuss the clips and develop a better understanding of the principles and, through time, we all come closer together.

Self-review has become massive. On the games that we've done, I would tend to have another look on the Monday and there is a self-review form for the referee that has a box for the TMO to comment.

Do you ever have any problems with the technology?

The systems we have in place are very reliable now. When we introduced the microphone communication system some years ago, initially we had some problems at some grounds but that has all been sorted out. Everybody accepts that getting the right decision is the most important thing.

How does TMO officiating differ from on-field officiating?

It's a lot more relaxed. There's not half as much physical training as for the referees.

Thoughts on the head mounted camera?

Recently Sky Sports have introduced the ref camera – a head mounted camera which gives a referee's perspective on the game. I'm personally not sure what the ref cameras actually add. I think in some ways they're too close. The angles quite often aren't what you expect them to be as they're often not looking at the right thing. I can't remember actually using the ref camera for a decision. It's also potentially dangerous. I think the referees in general prefer the chest camera.

Does the 'big screen' in the stadium affect the outcome of decisions?

Yes it does. There are some that are difficult to see depending upon where they are positioned in the stadium. Those that don't have them are beginning to realise that they're missing out, because the crowd doesn't get to share in the reviews. Newcastle is a nightmare because of where its positioned.

How does the 'big screen' in the stadium affect your decision-making?

When you know there isn't a big screen you tend to take a few more seconds to think through what you're going to say because you're translating it for everyone, but it doesn't affect your decision.

References

[1] Surujlal, J. & Jordan, D. B. (2013). Goal line technology in soccer: Are referees ready for technology in decision making? *African Journal for Physical, Health Education, Recreation and Dance, 19,* 245–57.

[2] Halmarick, A. (2002). *Television match official decision analysis for Super 12 rugby union 2002 season.* Australian Rugby.

[3] Lorains, M., Ball, K., & MacMahon, C. (2013). Expertise differences in a video decision-making task: Speed influences on performance. *Psychology of Sport and Exercise, 14,* 293–7.

[4] Borooah, V. K. (2014). Upstairs and downstairs: The imperfection of cricket's decision review system. *Journal of Sports Economics* (in press).

[5] Mahmood, T., Ahmed, S. O., Nayyer, S. H., & Swaleh, M. H. (2012). A-Eye: Automating the role of the third umpire in the game of cricket. *Expert Systems with Applications, 39,* 12280–9.

[6] Singh Bal, B., & Dureja, G. (2012). Hawk Eye: A logical innovative technology use in sports for effective decision making. *Sport Science Review, 21,* 107–119.

[7] Collins, H., & Evans, R. (2008). You cannot be serious! Public understanding of technology with special reference to "Hawk-Eye". *Public Understanding of Science, 17,* 283–308.

[8] Mather, G. (2008). Perceptual uncertainty and line-call challenges in professional tennis. *Proceedings of the Royal Society B, 275,* 1645–51.

[9] Abramitzky, R., Einav, L., Kolkowitz, S., & Mill, R. (2012). On the optimality of line call challenges in professional tennis. *International Economic Review, 53,* 939–63.

[10] Scheer, J. K., Ansorge, C. J., & Howard, J. (1983). Judging bias induced by viewing contrived videotapes: A function of selected psychological variables. *Journal of Sport Psychology, 5,* 427–37.

[11] Leveaux, R. (2010). Facilitating referee's decision making in sport via the application of technology. *Communications of the IBIMA,* 2010.

[12] Leveaux, R. (2012). 2012 Olympic Games decision making technologies for taekwondo competition. *Communications of the IBIMA,* 2012.

[13] Mackenzie, S. H., & Kerr, J. H. (2012). Head-mounted cameras and stimulated recall in qualitative sport research. *Qualitative Research in Sport, Exercise and Health, 4,* 51–61.

[14] Gilis, B., Weston, M., Helsen, W., Junge, A., & Dvorak, J. (2006). Interpretation and application of the laws of the game in football incidents leading to player injuries. *International Journal of Sport Psychology, 37,* 121–38.

9

SELECTION, TRAINING AND EVALUATION OF PERFORMANCE

Introduction

The selection, training and method of evaluating performance in officiating are critical for referees' performance quality. This chapter will review work that addresses some appropriate approaches to each of these tasks. The most up-to-date research and state-of-the-art in training and evaluation systems will be presented, focusing on different types of officiating. This chapter has been placed towards the end of the book as it will reflect the training implications raised in the preceding chapters and bring many of the issues together. It will cover the selection and recruiting of officials (from volunteers to developing elites), illustrate different training systems and present evaluation systems by showing methods of assessing effectiveness in officials and possible performance declines.

Selection and recruiting of officials

The selection and recruiting of sports officials is sport-dependent and differs between sport associations and even between regions. Generally, every person can become a sports official, with the only requirements being at least 14 years of age in most sports and being a member of a club. In most sports there are two broad categories of recruits: junior officials, who are in charge of junior sports officiating, and adults who frequently follow their own children's involvement in the respective sport. Very few sport associations require aspiring sports officials to provide evidence of having been active as an athlete in the sport they now would like to officiate. For instance, in horse dressage, aspiring sports officials have to have won medals as athletes on the level below the one they want to officiate. Therefore, as judges move higher in their licence level, their expertise level as athletes also needs to be higher. When these basic requirements are met, aspiring sports officials can sign up for basic courses, which are mostly weekend courses, after which they have to pass theoretical and practical tests. As they move higher in their licence level, further courses and examinations need to be taken, differing in amount and content, depending on the sport. In some sports additional fitness tests are required as some sports are characterised by high physical demands (see also Chapter 3 on physical demands in officiating).

The recruiting of new sports officials is mostly based on advertisements on the homepage of sport associations, in clubs or at schools. The International Football Association (FIFA) has put together regulations and recommendations to assist their member associations and match officials with their respective duties, such as recruiting new officials or retaining them.[1] Most sports have difficulties finding enough sports officials, which is why not much focus is put on specific requirements needed to become a sports official, as long as there is interest. To attract people, some sport associations provide the opportunity of having access to First League games and competitions as a spectator if regular officiating is shown. The recruiting of expert sports officials is based on officiating performance as well as theoretical and practical examinations. If a rookie sports official is selected as being talented, he/she will be closely monitored and evaluated, with mentors (mostly former expert sports officials) training and supporting them. The pathway to an elite sports official is usually quite long – for example, an average of 16 years for soccer referees to reach the FIFA list[2] – since aspiring referees have no possibility of skipping a level in their career progression based on officiating skill. Some associations have proposed the recruitment of former elite players and a reduction in the number of years it takes to reach a high level.[3, 4] This so-called fast-track system is in line with findings that indicate positive implications for transfer of processing skill during these role transitions, such as players who become referees, as outlined in Chapter 2.

Once recruited, however, an additional problem is the retention of sports officials. Retention is defined as being successful in retaining the provision of services of sports officials from one season to the next. Especially at the grassroots level, associations have to manage an increasing number of dropouts (e.g., DFB, German Football Association, 2012, or the Australian Sports Commission, 2004). In a report prepared for the Australian Sports Commission, 142 sports officials of five different sports were interviewed on recruitment and retention of sports officials. The results showed that there are significant problems with retention at the grassroots level. Different reasons were identified, such as inadequate resources and facilities, poor integration of the operation of sports governing organisations, poor feedback and abuse by coaches and spectators.[5] Abuse by spectators has even gone so far that referees are faced with life-threatening attacks – for instance, the death of a Dutch assistant referee after an attack by teenage players.[6] Titlebaum and co-workers[7] reported that severe problems with recruitment and retention also exist for high school and college officiating in the USA. Although many issues cannot be controlled by sports associations, factors related to sports official's sources of stress could be a starting point. These include performance concerns, time pressure and lack of recognition. In their study they propose strategies to help recruit new officials and ways to retain current officials. The resulting framework for a successful programme includes eight points[7] (page 107):

- market the job
- set standards for officials under consideration to be hired
- continually evaluate officials and the programme
- set up mentoring programmes
- create incentives for staff members
- create a job structure where students can advance within the programme
- set policies of how games will be assigned
- hold fans, spectators and officials accountable for their behaviour during an event.

The abovementioned aspects on the retention of sports officials mostly contain negative experiences of sports officials and how to overcome these. However, one can also focus on the positive aspects of officiating and examine the reasons why officials continue their job despite abuse and other stress factors. It has been shown that social interaction seems to be crucial to officiating retention.[8] From their findings, the authors suggest that sports officials seem to use social interaction as a positive reinforcement and a tool for re-framing punishers. Through interactions with other sports officials, they seem to learn and understand abuse as part of the sport system and culture. Therefore, detecting aspects why officials continue to officiate and develop strategies based on this knowledge might be another approach to retaining sports officials in their job.

Training systems

Chapters 3 and 7 described the physical and psychological demands put on sports officials during games and competitions. In order to be able to cope with these demands and perform at a high level of officiating, training systems must be developed to support the education of expert sport officials. The expert performance approach by Ericsson and co-workers[9] proposes an increase in deliberate practice activities; however, this mostly resulted from studies on musicians and sport athletes. Transferring this approach to more cognitive tasks such as judgement and decision making of sports officials would implicate an increase in officiating experience. Officiating a high number of games or competitions, accompanied by officiating coaches providing constructive feedback, may provide lasting experiences in officiating. However, since there are limits in the number of games to referee, an alternative way of training might be to use video training, which will be discussed later.

Basic training

The most basic requirement in officiating is knowledge of the rules and laws of the sport, which is referred to as declarative knowledge or rule book knowledge.

In general, aspiring sports officials are equipped with materials including the law book (e.g., in soccer or rugby union), rule book (e.g., in basketball) or code book (e.g., in gymnastics), accompanied by commentaries and videos explaining these. To give some examples, gymnastics judges need to know 700–800 skills, the racing rules of sailing include 91 rules with several sub-rules, and volleyball, ice hockey and basketball referees need to know 30, 35 and 59 hand signals, respectively, in addition to the rules. Basic training then includes the mere study of the written rules, becoming familiar with the specific rule system and getting to know the terminology. Weekend workshops bring together sports officials to practise their declarative knowledge, observe and discuss athletes' performance on video clips and learn about new rules and their applications.

Training on the field or in the gym

The implementation of the rules is referred to as procedural knowledge. Several attempts have been made to develop training tools focusing on different aspects of a referee's task and therefore training and enhancing procedural knowledge. In general, the development of training tools should focus on the demands, key decisions or typical errors as identified in Chapters 4 and 5. A distinction should also be made between physically demanding officiating such as in soccer, as well as less physically demanding officiating such as in gymnastics. In sports requiring more physical activity by the sports official, training should mimic the on-field demands and comprise aerobic aspects accordingly. Training for physical fitness is mostly not standardised in sports associations. Referees usually train by themselves with their own training schedule in order to meet the requirements imposed on them during fitness tests. Referees report that their training involves aerobic training sessions such as running, swimming and cycling, as well as speed/sprint training and strength programme sessions (for an overview see Blake et al.[10] for Gaelic games referees and MacMahon et al.[2] for soccer referees).

Attempts have been made to scientifically develop training programs to improve refereeing-specific aerobic metabolism. For instance, Krustrup and Bangsbo[11] had Danish elite soccer referees perform a 12-week training programme consisting of interval running with short and long intervals. The results revealed that, after this intermittent exercise training, referees significantly improved their performance concerning repeated shuttle running, time to exhaustion, heart rates and blood lactate concentration. In addition, game-relevant activities were taken into account, showing that although the referees did not increase their total distance covered during a game, the distance covered during high intensity running was increased. However, a crucial aspect of refereeing is the accuracy of decisions. Although not directly shown in this study, the mean distance from infringements in the attacking zones was significantly less after the training than before, which might be an indicator of keeping up with play and achieving the best viewing position to make accurate judgements of fast-moving players (see Chapter 4). Similar results of an improvement in aerobic metabolism were found with Belgian referees after sixteen months of specific training.[12] More studies are needed in this field, however, to examine the impact of exercise capacity on judgemental errors in officiating and, more specifically, the effect of fatigue on cognitive judgements (for more information see Chapter 3).

Independent of physical fitness, high volumes of deliberate practice in relevant activities to improve specific officiating skills as well as maximisation of officiating actual competition (officiating experience) should be obtained to emphasise the influence of context and realistic scenarios. These principles have been summarised for decision-making training in athletes[13] and can be similarly used as guidelines for sports officials. Figure 9.1 presents an example of how this decision-training model can be transferred and adapted to the training of decisions on fouls by soccer referees.

Sport associations and their officiating coaches should follow these principles when designing, running and assessing training activities. These can then be implemented in training camps, workshops, controlled games and 'shadowing', where a novice official follows an experienced official.

However, training on the field or in the gym not only needs to focus on a sports officials' task, but can also mimic a player's or athlete's perspective. As illustrated in Chapter 2, sports officials often show impressive motor experiences as athletes in their history profiles. Since several situations on the field require quick and accurate perception, putting themselves into the situation of the

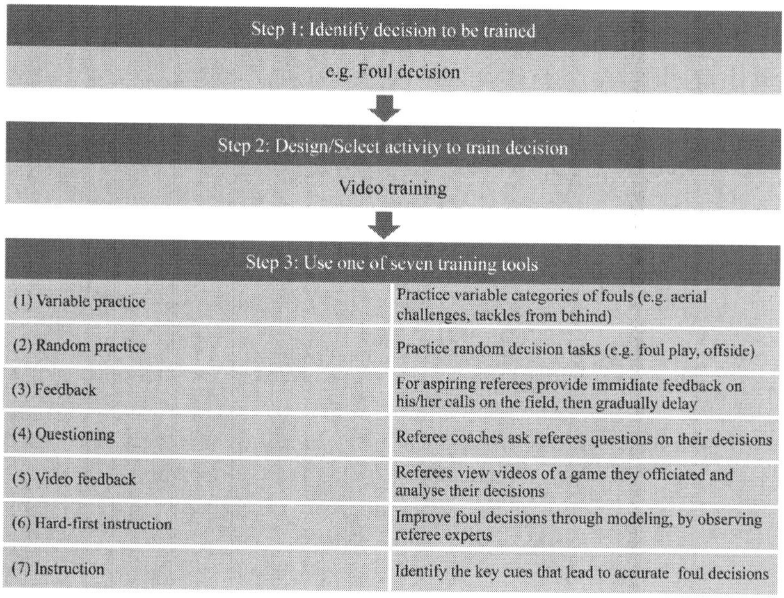

Step 1: Identify decision to be trained	
e.g. Foul decision	

Step 2: Design/Select activity to train decision	
Video training	

Step 3: Use one of seven training tools	
(1) Variable practice	Practice variable categories of fouls (e.g. aerial challenges, tackles from behind)
(2) Random practice	Practice random decision tasks (e.g. foul play, offside)
(3) Feedback	For aspiring referees provide immidiate feedback on his/her calls on the field, then gradually delay
(4) Questioning	Referee coaches ask referees questions on their decisions
(5) Video feedback	Referees view videos of a game they officiated and analyse their decisions
(6) Hard-first instruction	Improve foul decisions through modeling, by observing referee experts
(7) Instruction	Identify the key cues that lead to accurate foul decisions

FIGURE 9.1 Modified decision-training model by Vickers[13] applied to soccer referees.

athletes might help the sports officials with their decisions. For instance, in ball games the detection of fouls and violations is often complicated by the fact that players frequently set out to intentionally deceive the observer.[14] Therefore, one aspect of coaching referees in decision making is to guide their attention to the deceptive behaviour of athletes by self-experiencing the situation (see Box 9.1).

BOX 9.1 STUDY ON DECEPTIVE MOVEMENTS IN SOCCER

In an intervention study with 40 expert soccer players,[15] specific motor and visual experiences of participants were manipulated by teaching the motor learning group to fake fouls and having the visual group watch the training. Over four weeks, with two training sessions per week, the motor group was asked to fake fouls in different categories. In one-on-one situations, one attacker in possession of the ball had to try to get past the defender who, in turn, was asked to try to get to the ball. As soon as the two players made body contact, the offensive player was asked to fake (simulate) having been fouled. The foul categories represented typical scenarios during games with, for example, players pretending to have been kicked or tripped by the defender's feet or using the contact of the opponent's upper body to simulate a body check (see Figure 9.2). The visual group attended the training sessions, watched and rated the motor group on the quality of their faked fouls and heard the feedback given to them. A taxonomy of behaviours associated with deceptive and non-deceptive intentions was used to provide appropriate feedback,[14] such as temporal contiguity, ballistic contiguity and contact consistency. In order to test the effect of this training on referee-specific decision making, video tests were conducted before and after the training intervention. The video clips matched the foul categories that had been trained. Participants were asked to decide whether the situation in the video clip represented no foul, a foul, a foul with a yellow card or a foul with a red card. The results revealed that the groups did not significantly enhance their decision-making accuracy. However, the motor group showed the strongest post-test retention test improvement compared to the visual group and a control group (who participated in the video tests only), although not significantly. Concerning decision time, all three groups became significantly faster in the video test, with the visual group showing the biggest improvement. This effect of visual experience was additionally supported by the findings that participants with a higher frequency of watching soccer on TV or on the field and with a higher amount of accumulated visual experience in years made significantly faster and more accurate decisions respectively.[16] Generalisations of these results with referees need to be conducted in order to give clear evidence-based implications. In sum, however, the findings provide a basis for a different approach to referee training, in that decision-making performance of such fouls and violations can be trained on the field by having referees watch these scenarios in a real environment.

(continued)

(continued)

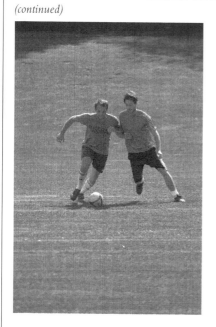

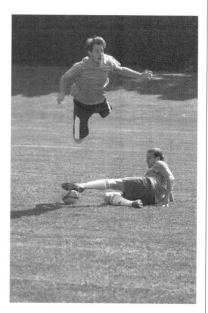

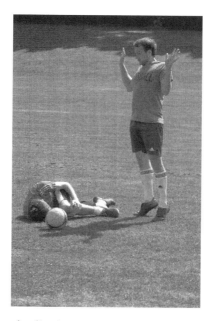

FIGURE 9.2 Learning the dive in soccer.

Competitive sport is generally accompanied by a high amount of acute stress due to performance errors, environmental conditions such as crowd noise or cheating athletes. Since acute stress can inhibit psychological as well as somatic processes during sporting competitions (e.g., attention, concentration, arousal), coping effectively with these stressful situations is crucial for high quality performance. In a study with 137 skilled basketball referees, Anshel and Weinberg[17] examined coping styles and their use in different stressful situations. The results indicated significant differences between coping styles as a function of the type of stressor. For instance, avoidance coping (e.g., ignoring the coach/athlete, quickly continuing play, concentrating on the game) was most prevalent for 'coping with player abuse' and 'arguing with coaches', whereas approach coping (e.g., calling a technical foul, trying to 'sell' the call, answering politely) was more often used for 'abuse by the coach'. Training for sports officials could include this aspect of coping with stressful events. Since it is difficult to teach coping strategies that do not fall within a person's style, a possible approach in sports officiating could be to train different adaptive coping strategies that the referee can then use to his/her disposal. However, the efficacy of such training interventions awaits further investigation.

Training off the field: video-based training

Since there are physical limits to how much can be trained on the field, training programmes focusing on the cognitive demands of officiating are recommended. Similar to on-the-field training, training tools should zoom in on the demands, key decisions or typical errors in officiating. For instance, video training methods combined with appropriate feedback have been shown to enhance offside decisions[18–20] and decision making in potential foul situations in soccer.[21, 22] In a study with rugby referees, a video-based training programme was designed to develop referees' shared mental models.[23] Referees studied training tapes consisting of different sets of tackles viewed over a six-week period. The videos were taken from real game referee perspectives to adapt to the complexity and dynamics of the naturalistic environment. The results showed that the lowest ranked referees in particular significantly improved their correct decisions after the training. Consequently, the English Rugby Football Union have employed this training into their educational programme to train accurate decision making, identify and train problem areas in refereeing and discuss new interpretations of tackle situations. For an example of decision-making training for soccer referees, see Box 9.2.

There are several challenges in developing video-based training:

1. Choosing appropriate video clips that offer different levels of difficulty concerning the correct decision.
2. Video clips should provide a similar point of view to that which the on-field or on-court official might have.

> # BOX 9.2 STUDY ON DECISION-MAKING TRAINING FOR SOCCER REFEREES
>
> In a study on decision making in potential foul situations in soccer, players as well as expert referees participated in a video-based training intervention with seven training sessions, each consisting of 22 videos.[22] Participants were asked to observe the videos and decide as quickly as possible between the options foul or no foul. If the option foul was chosen, further decisions had to be made concerning the type of sanction (free kick, free kick and yellow card, free kick and red card). If participants had correctly decided (including the correct sanction in the foul decision), they received the feedback 'That's correct' or 'That's wrong' in the case of a wrong decision. Results showed that all participants significantly enhanced their decision accuracy by an average of seven per cent (three decisions) when immediate feedback after each video clip was given. In another study,[24] basketball referees were instructed to focus on defensive fouls. Although the referees did not show significant improvement in the video-based infraction detection task, the study showed that focusing in more detail on different abilities such as the detection of fouls and violations can enhance the decision making of sports officials.

3.   When providing feedback on the sports officials' performance in the video training, the 'correct' call needs to be determined in advance. But how is this accomplished? The ambiguity and fuzziness of foul situations need to be acknowledged in order to provide sensitive evaluations. The fact that context is usually absent in these video clips needs to be taken into account.

In general, focus can be put on different aspects of the movement or situation to be judged, taking into account the rules and codes of the different sports. In order to provide accurate feedback, video clips should be judged by experts as well as performing detailed video analyses. In that way, subjective measures can be combined with objective measures such as angles and height.

Performance evaluation

Evaluation systems in officiating are crucial for assessing the performance of sports officials. Considering the high impact sports officials can have on game and competition outcomes, either on an economical or emotional basis, performance should be transparent and judgements and decisions should be as fair and accurate as possible. Depending on the sport, different evaluation systems exist, focusing on task-specific performance as well as physical performance, in cases of physically demanding officiating. Physical fitness is regularly evaluated, especially in ball games, including for instance the assessment of endurance on the one hand and speed on the other hand (for an example of the FIFA fitness test, see Chapter 3).

Task-specific performance measures in ball games such as soccer, basketball, handball and ice hockey are taken with an observation system in which expert referee coaches regularly watch referees during their games and judge them on different aspects characteristic of good referee performance (see Figure 9.3 for an example in basketball). These characteristics differ as a function of sport type, but generally performance is rated on the implementation of the game rules (e.g., understanding of the game, foul situations, penalties) and on personal impressions (e.g., referee appearance, positioning, game management). Points are given according to the performance in different categories and then summed up to a final performance measure with higher points representing better performance. The resulting protocols/evaluations are then used for feedback, but also for the determination of referee scheduling for important games.

Performance measures in technical sports such as trampoline are often taken from the theory examinations (see Figure 9.4 for an example in basketball). These include questions on rule-based knowledge and the analysis of videotaped trampoline routines, similar to the demands at real competitions. The results of the theoretical tests are used to determine judging performance and, consequently, decide whether a judge can proceed to a higher judging level/licence.

Although most sports associations apply evaluations in their education, almost none have externally validated their evaluation systems. Since the officials' demands are not necessarily observable or captured by specific criteria, it is even more difficult to find evaluation systems that cover all aspects in a transparent manner. At this point, collaborations between researchers and practitioners seem crucial in order to exchange expertise in the respective fields. One such approach has been used

BIG V

VJBL

REFEREE EVALUATION GAME REPORT

EVALUATOR		GAME / ROUND NO.	9	DATE	
REFEREE		UMPIRE		UMPIRE	

This report is for the official whose name is in bold and underlined.

HOME	SPBA	AWAY	Latrobe	VENUE	SPBA
GAME RATING	DIFFICULT	AVERAGE	Y	EASY	
League:	Big V	Division:	D-1	Male/Female:	Men

1. FOULS	Score out of 20	16
2. VIOLATIONS	Score out of 10	8
3. MECHANICS & AOR	Score out of 10	7
4. POE & RULES APPLICATION	Score out of 10	7
DECISIONS & JUDGEMENT	Score out of 60	38
1. PLAYER/COACH COMMUNICATION	Score out of 20	15
2. TEAMWORK	Score out of 10	8
3. HANDLING OF NO CALLS	Score out of 10	8
4. LEADERSHIP	Score out of 10	8
GAME MANAGEMENT	Score out of 50	39
TOTAL SCORE	Score out of 100	77
VBRA Panel	BAND RANGE	80 -85
VBRA Panel	BAND RANGE	75 - 80
VBRA Panel Other	BAND RANGE	70 - 75

1. TOTAL SCORES SHOULD GENERALLY BE WITHIN THE BAND RANGE RELEVANT TO THE OFFICIALS PANEL.
2 IF THE OFFICIAL PERFORMS ABOVE OR BELOW WHAT IS EXPECTED OF THEIR RANGE. BOTH THE SCORE AND WRITTEN REPORT MUST REFLECT THAT PERFORMANCE
3. REFER TO THE ATTACHED SCORE CRITERIA AS A GUIDE FOR SCORING RELATIVE TO PERFORMANCE

1.&2. FOULS/VIOLATIONS (INCL-ADV/DIS)
Charge /block - ref the defence, and get some consistency on that "window". There were two here that I would have liked you to knock down more accurately.

3. MECHANICS & AREAS OF RESPONSIBIL
No issues noticeable, but I do feel you could be more mobile in lead

4. POE & RULES APPLICATION
CH/BL, as mentioned

1. PLAYER/COACH COMMUNICATION
Pretty good, but both coaches could have been controlled a little more firmly. Run over to them when the were yelling to stop the uglyness, then explain and warn.

2. TEAMWORK
The pregame must have worked and the start of the game showed it. This was an absolute strength - you were both one the same line from the toss.

3. HANDLING OF NO CALLS
Talk- but late on these. The one line explanation will help here. A strength - you let them play and called what was required almost perfectly.

4. LEADERSHIP
Exhibited plenty from the start - just the coach dialogue to improve on. Don't let yelling matches continue - stop them fast, politely and firmly.

A. AREAS TO WORK ON
1. Charge Block - get that window right. Always ref that defence. 2. Management - Both coaches yelled a number of times and got quite aggressive. While it didn't effect too much, it looked ugly. Get over to them so it's not as public, explain and then instruct them to ask politely next time without the agro.

B. TOTAL SCORE PERFORMANCE
You both hit the court as a tight unit brilliantly, and we had a great 1 point thriller because of it. Your teamwork and consistency really added to this game, and I have scored you outside the norm because of it. Errors were minimal, management with the players excellent, the line you called for the teams perfect - and they showed how they appreciated it with their play. Well done - be proud of this one.

C. SCORE BENCH & VENUE ISSUES
Nil

FIGURE 9.3 Example of a basketball referee evaluation report.

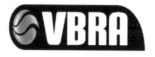

KNOX REFEREES AGM EXAMINATION
ANSWERS ARE EITHER TRUE OR FALSE

1. On a throw in from the end line, it is legal to throw the ball over the top of the backboard.

2. An unsportsmanlike foul must always involve contact with an opposing player.

3. A Coach can request for a time out to be less than one minute.

4. A4 commits an unsportsmanlike foul against B5, after which Team "A" is awarded a time out. When play resumes, B5 is not successful in either of his free throw attempts. Before the remaining throw in resulting from the A4 foul, the coach of Team "A" requests another time out. The time out shall be granted.

5. A4 in his backcourt attempts a fast break pass to A5 in his frontcourt. B6 jumps from his frontcourt, catches the ball while airborne and lands straddling the centre line. B6 then dribbles into his backcourt. This is legal play.

6. For a referee to determine if a player has travelled, the referee should first establish which foot is the pivot foot.

7. A4 is straddling the centre line. He receives the ball from A5 who is in the backcourt. A4 then passes the ball back to A5 in the backcourt. This is legal play.

8. You should always check the score sheet or Sportingpulse before the start of a game.

9. A4 is dribbling the ball in his backcourt and ends his dribble while straddling the centre line. A4 then passes the ball to A5 who is straddling the centre line. This is a violation by "A" team.

Make sure that you have given an answer to every question. If you are uncertain about your answer, go with your feeling and put what you think it should be.

If you have changed an answer make sure you put a large cross through the incorrect answer and then shade in and circle the correct one.

FIGURE 9.4 Example of a basketball referee examination form.

by Anshel[25] by developing and externally validating a new observational rating instrument, the behaviourally anchored rating scale for assessing the competencies of basketball referees (BARS-BR). Two groups with varying degrees and types of experience and expertise in basketball officiating developed a rating scale consisting of thirteen categories, with three behavioural examples each. The categories were the following: (1) mastery of rules; (2) effective on-court verbal communication; (3) effective on-court non-verbal communication; (4) proper mechanics; (5) effective off-court communication; (6) high fitness level; (7) professional on-court presentation; (8) actively contributes to games; (9) tries to improve own standard/ skills; (10) uses critical feedback; (11) interacts effectively with partner; (12) maintains credibility; and (13) engages in proper mental and physical pre-game preparation.

The BARS-BR was then externally validated and proven to be effective based on statistical comparisons of highly skilled and novice male and female basketball referees.

Researchers have also attempted to combine the different findings and provide an overview of the complexity of explaining the performances of sports officials. Guillén and Feltz[26] and Mascarenhas and co-workers[27] have developed models and frameworks focusing on different aspects. These include, for instance, knowledge and application of the rules, contextual judgement, personality, fitness, positioning and referee efficacy. A very interesting approach has been shown by Mascarenhas et al. in their study on rugby referees.[27] With the aim to identify a framework for referee training and selection, they developed the Cornerstones Performance Model of Refereeing which features four key areas:

- knowledge and application of laws/rules
- contextual judgement
- personality and management skills
- fitness, positioning and mechanics.

The whole model is overarched by the psychological characteristics of excellence, such as confidence, concentration and ambition. In interviews with expert groups, the usefulness of the model was confirmed and is now used (with further adaptations[28]) to develop rugby referees throughout England. Interestingly, the aspect of confidence, as described in the Cornerstones Performance Model of Refereeing, was highlighted in a new model for soccer referees by Guillén and Feltz.[26] According to this conceptual model of referee efficacy, the extent to which referees believe in their capacity to perform successfully (refficacy) is hypothesised to influence, amongst other factors, also referee performance. Given that this model was developed based on interviews with referee experts, it is still lacking empirical evidence by testing and extending it in the real-world environment. From a physical perspective, a notational analysis study investigating the in-game movement patterns completed by rugby union referees resulted in the JAM intermittent fitness test.[29] This test replicates the movement patterns required in the game with bouts of walking, jogging, running and sprinting, each linked by turns that replicate the frequency of changes in running speed that referees experience while officiating. Thus, different interesting approaches exist to develop models explaining, predicting and evaluating referee performance.

Official's call (1)

Jacqui Jashari

Introduction

My experiences officiating at Commonwealth Games, World Championships and many Test Matches and then coaching and mentoring umpires at an international, national and state level have given me a good insight into what it is like when being assessed and actually being the assessor.

The notion that the pathway to an elite sports official averages 16 years seems valid from my experience. What you do to stay at that level, however, can become more challenging than the original journey. The question is: What is the difference between a good umpire and a great umpire? Is it being in the right place at the right time? Getting the opportunities? Is it commitment, physical and mental attributes or just plain talent?

It was a natural progression for me to begin to coach and mentor umpires. I valued the people who coached and mentored me and understood from the start the huge impact they would have on my officiating aspirations and where I wanted to go. It is important to ensure the relationship is right between coaches and mentors and the officials with whom they are involved. If the relationship is not right there is no value to either party. There is also a difference between a coach and a mentor; it can be the same person, but that person needs to know which hat they are wearing and when.

Selection

Officials move in and out of the umpire continuum for many reasons – Recruit, Retain and Reward has been the mantra for a long time. Many sports have programmes based around this that are successful and continue to be so. Recruiting is important, but it is what happens to the officials once the sport has them that is even more influential. The examples in the chapter demonstrate this through the data gathered, and so it is not a surprise. Support structures that surround entry level officials through to the elite level are the key.

It is great to have the numbers, and a big group of officials, but the quality, commitment and knowledge is just as important. Focusing on the positive aspects of officiating is paramount for retention and development. Educating officials around the tools needed to deal with any negative issues and providing training on the application of the rules to the game and in context is crucial.

Training systems

Officials need to train to umpire. They can certainly be the fittest person off the court, but it does not make them 'match ready'. Mostly it is the 'quality' and not the 'quantity' of training that officials need to focus on. What is it they need to be doing when they are out on the court? What are the areas that have been identified for improvement? The deliberate practice approach is effective and it has shaped my officiating, particularly at the elite level.

Fitness in netball officiating is critical. The umpire needs to be as fit as – if not fitter than – the players in order to keep up with play. They must have the ability to change direction quickly, communicate to players through voice and hand signals and maintain a high level of concentration within each fifteen minute quarter.

It can be difficult to train umpires to get the 'feel' for the game. Some have it naturally and others have to work very hard at it. There needs to be a good mix of match experience, attending training sessions with players, so umpires can learn what the players are capable of within the rules of the game, off-court fitness and video analysis. Communication and interaction with players and coaches in a training environment also plays a huge part in an umpire's training. This communication begins to build the mutual respect that is required, allowing opportunities after the match and often after the heat of the game to discuss different points of view.

Performance evaluation

Assessment and evaluation systems should be developed dependent on the sport's requirements. There is no one size fits all, considering you have the 'mobile umpire' and the 'technical judge'.

My experience has been that, with a comprehensive theoretical and large practical component, assessment is by numbers or terms and examination-based. Sports should be cautious with the true examination-based tests as often umpires can demonstrate skill out on the court but have difficulty writing or articulating responses. This chapter addresses the psychological characteristics of excellence well.

When assessing or evaluating, it is important to understand why an official made either an incorrect or correct decision and the factors that had an impact on this. Were they in the right position at the right time? Did they look at the right time? Did they process what they were seeing? Did they apply the correct rule to the scenario and could they process the multiple actions that they saw? Invasion sports require the umpire to see all the players most of the time and make assessments. The methods of assessing and evaluating umpires need to take into consideration all of the questions above.

There needs to be flexibility in learning styles and evaluation process for officials, as often this is a barrier to umpires remaining in the sport.

Conclusion

This chapter is a great read and provides those involved as coaches and/or mentors with an opportunity to challenge the way they train and evaluate the officials they work with.

Official's call (2)

Tony Parker

Introduction

This chapter centres predominantly around soccer and other field sports where fitness to keep up with play is important. I am a qualified official in squash, cricket and table tennis, all of which have different requirements for officials. While all three require good hearing and eyesight, fitness and athleticism is not important, except for the quick mobility required of a cricket umpire to move to the correct position to judge run outs and avoid being hit by the ball!

Training

Of the three sports with which I am involved, table tennis is the easiest. There are very few difficult rules and the game is really in need only of a scorer. The only problem area is the legality of the serve. I'm not aware of any examinations. Experienced umpires just mentor new people and then appoint them to matches.

Most umpires are retired players at all levels from County down to club, and to become a club umpire requires no special qualifications. League umpires are required to pass a written examination which covers all possible events that require an umpire's decision including some situations which are so contrived that I've never come across them as an umpire, player or spectator. If an umpire wants to move up to County matches, a member of the Umpire Association will meet them, arrange for them to umpire a match and assess their performance in one or two matches before they will be appointed to County matches. As virtually all umpires are ex-players, they are aware of the role of the umpire.

Skills

Of the three sports for which I am qualified, my main experience is as a squash referee where I progressed right to the top as a World Referee and am now a World Referee Assessor. The rules of the game are quite straightforward but interpretation is the most important aspect. Only a thorough understanding of the tactics of the players, which vary considerably between club players and top professionals, is needed to be a proficient referee at each level. Anyone who has not played the game to a reasonable level would find acquiring the relevant skills very difficult.

Incentives and career spans

There is a shortage of referees at all levels from top World Referees down to local, club and County. There are two main reasons for this shortage: they are not paid for their services and they have other priorities in life.

Regarding pay, referees even at World Championships are paid only expenses of travel and accommodation and food. Officials who would be ideally qualified to become referees such as retired professional players won't go into refereeing because they need to earn money from coaching or another squash-related activity that provides an income.

The current age of most referees is 50 and above and many carry on into their 70s because there are no younger referees coming through to take their place. The other reason good younger prospective referees are not around is life priorities. They probably have limited free time through a combination of still playing regularly, family commitments and maybe limited holidays from their employment. England Squash and Racquetball (ESR), however, still actively tries to recruit referees initially through County Associations. Once they have attained the lowest qualification, ESR arranges an annual conference over one weekend when all referees are invited, all expenses paid (including hotel) and senior referees give talks on selected topics. These conferences are well attended with 50–60 referees attending each year.

Qualification systems

The lowest qualification in squash and racquetball, termed Club Grade, is awarded after the candidate has attended a course given by an approved instructor and completed a written examination which they can complete in their own time and is open book. This gives them status within their club.

The next stage is County Grade, which can be awarded by the County Association to those referees who wish to progress and is awarded to all referees who show they are competent to referee County matches. The next grade is Tournament level, which is awarded when a County referee has had a minimum of three assessments over a year. They are then qualified to referee at National Competitions in the early rounds up to the quarter final stages. This level of appointment is made by the referee co-ordinator from ESR based on the County's recommendation.

Specially designed assessment forms are used for promotion from County to Tournament Grade and only National Grade referees can undertake these assessments.

For promotion to National Grade, the highest grade within any country, whilst the same type of assessment form is used, candidates must achieve a performance with fewer mistakes and in more difficult matches. As with County to Tournament 3, competent assessments are required and from more than one assessor of which at least one must be from a higher grade referee.

The next step for the best of any country's referees is Regional Grade which, for British referees, is Europe. Regional referees can be put forward by their region to become World Squash Referees. Different assessment forms are used for Regional and World referees, with more detail and a greater requirement for competent control and management of matches between the World top players.

Whilst there is no minimum time a referee can be considered for promotion from their existing grade, the average is two years at each grade. However, exceptional candidates can progress more quickly while others require more experience. Some are happy to remain at their grades, not wishing to take on the stress of higher profile matches but are invaluable in the early rounds of tournaments.

Mentorship and the role of the official

All referees at all levels are encouraged to find a mentor who would be at a higher grade than they are. The governing bodies do not appoint mentors as it is important that the referee and mentor have a good relationship and this is best achieved when the candidate chooses their mentor.

Decisions at all levels when it comes to players getting in each others' way are subjective, although within the rules. Some players are more disposed to expressing disagreement and the management and control of these players is an essential experience top referees have to gain. Referees have great powers in issuing penalties when necessary, from just a warning to a stroke to a game or even the match. Obscene language and gestures are not tolerated and would certainly cost a player a game or even the whole match. Most sports have similar rules and player behaviour standards (e.g, rugby). So it makes me wonder why soccer referees have to put up with the player conduct so often seen on television.

Official's call (3)

Tom Lopes

Training, recruitment and progression

My experience with refereeing is that, once you got a taste for it, you wanted the top game and you had that confidence, there's nothing that can happen that you can't handle. In the old days you would have that confidence to know that there's nothing that can happen that you can't handle, and certainly that was from the preparation we received from practitioners who taught us how to do it. And you refine it on your own, and in your own particular style. Those days are pretty well gone. We're becoming more robotic where everything has to be the same.

The pathways are different now. If you look at a qualified high school official trying to move into the College ranks – you must go to the try-out camps that each of the college supervisors run for their conference. They're under game conditions and referees must pay to come to the camps, where they try-out and try to make their best impression. The problem is that there is not a whole lot of turnover, so the supervisors might only take three, four or five officials each year out of 60 to 80 to 100 trying out. It's extremely competitive. And with my supervisors and selectors, we will have a little scoping session, where they'll ask, "Tom, what are you looking for?" My answer is, "I'm not sure but I know it when I see it".

Often the guys who make it come from occupations where they can get away in the afternoons, such as education people and school administrators and the self-employed. NBA referees are employees. At all other levels in the USA, officials are independent contractors.

A cadet (new) official has to come to a class, usually twelve weeks, usually two hours a night, followed by testing on the particular rules they've been looking at each night. This is then followed by a written test one day in November on which they must score 84 out of 100, all yes/no questions. They then become partly certified where they take a floor test to learn mechanics, positioning, signals etc. This takes a season. Then the next year they're certified and they start out at the elementary school junior varsity level. They're then evaluated during their regular season games. There is just one certified level as an IAABO official and they have to earn their levels with their local boards and attend at least four of five board meetings through the year.

Mentoring

Mentors who are retired ex-officials selected by the board will go out, watch the game and sit with the young officials usually for about an hour after the game. They will look through the video, look at positioning, mechanics, body language – all the things that affect the referee's performance. The programme is really good because the referees feel that they have somebody to fall back on and have someone to give them some positive and critical feedback.

Reputation and development

All my staff of seventy officials at the college level are pretty much equal. But what makes one a little bit better than the other is when you walk in the gym and the coach is looking and says, "Oh, that's Tom Lopes. We know what we get in that package. He might not be any better than the rest of them, but we know what we'll get. He will communicate with us, he might make a mistake or two but we're comfortable with him." New kids come in and the coach's first comment is, "Who the hell is that new guy?" He might be better than me or the other two guys, but the coaches and we don't know him.

It's hard for the young guys. A good referee has that ability to communicate with the coach without being confrontational. This means things like using the one word that relaxes and calms the situation, being in the right position to make that call, showing good body language, being accurate with your decisions. The questions you need to ask are: Are you approachable or standoff-ish? Are your hands on your hips saying "Alright, try me"? These are the kind of things that may put an obstacle in your path. My suggestion for the younger guys is to find out what the veteran officials are using and saying, and try to incorporate these in your repertoire.

Top referees have an aura, a command, a presence. I would say that the top coaches relax when they see me. They know that the game is in good hands. They can relax and return to coaching and not have to worry about the officials. And the biggest thing they want is communication. Also, there's a crispness to the signals and calls of the top officials. When you blow the whistle, everyone knows what it is that has taken place. Basketball is probably the fastest sport to officiate. You need a combination of all these things to make it. At the lower levels you will get by on your communication skills.

Selection and assignment

Each of our IAABO boards has an assignor who picks from a pool of officials. These pools are typically freshman, junior varsity and varsity. The pools are decided on an evaluation basis each year to determine movement between categories. When I'm assigning varsity games I look at my varsity pool, knowing what sort of game it's going to be, and I appoint depending upon the difficulty of the game. There is no guidance on playing experience to become an official.

Officiating style

Those days where we had our own style are pretty much gone. We're becoming pretty robotic, where everything has to be the same. For example, in the National Football League (NFL) and the National Basketball Association (NBA) they have a defined staff, and either you do it this way or you don't have a job. In the NBA there are 17,000 officials and getting them on the same page is difficult. Also, in being a good official, you should look the part and your partners have a lot to do with it too.

Abuse

As far as abuse to officials goes, my philosophy is that you only hear what you need to hear. The worst people are the parents. The parents of 10–12-year-old children think they know everything. But you can't be reactive. There are ways to deal with it. Many high school games and college games have security available. Instead of making a scene, you walk over to security and say, "You see that person over there in the red jacket? I'd like them removed". This way you're not dealing with confrontation. There are pathways that you can use to make these things go away.

Mistakes

I tell my officials that they have got to admit their mistakes. If you've made a mistake, you have to own up to it and then you can move on and put it behind you. I can live with that, but I can't live with misapplying a rule. If you misapply a rule, that is a different matter. It's going to happen to every official. Somewhere along the line a decision that you make is going to turn the tide of a game or cost somebody a game. But you have to suck it in and learn from that mistake, because it's going to make you a better official in the long run.

We also tell the officials that it's okay to admit "I blew that call". Then you say, I'm going to work harder and try to be better. Being a good official starts with getting the calls right.

Social interaction

Social interaction is important for our guys because each board is kind of like a club where they are a member, and I think that camaraderie helps to keep them together. We lose officials due to age or as they move out of state, or some who have big aspirations but don't progress as they would wish so they get frustrated and leave. Our retention is pretty good. We're all together as a group so it's almost like a fraternity, and I think that helps to keep us together. We have a few who feel they never had a chance and they leave, but only the minority.

Decision making and deception

The research on diving in soccer is a good topic. In basketball we make a yearly video that highlights areas of concern and, in these areas of concern, we have plays that show 'flopping' (where the defender falls over to deceive the official related to the contact that has occurred). We provide ideas on ways to handle it. According to the rules there are a few ways of dealing with it. One is if a player is attempting to deceive the official they should be given an unsporting technical foul. Or you just leave them on the floor, don't blow the whistle and don't make any suggestions. You can also call a block and tell them to 'knock it off'. We are trying to get everyone on the same page in dealing with this. It's a work in progress and it is a hot topic.

Evaluation

As a supervisor, every play of every game is 'cut out' for me so I can say, "At 3 minutes 35 you had a block/charge call. Let's look at it." And I'll ask, "What were you looking at?" In fact my officials have to give me two plays that they think were questionable during their game and we'll both look at them the next day. And there may be ones that I ask them to look at as well.

I'll ask them, "First, were there any incidents that I have to be aware of? Was there a fight, was there a technical foul? Second, how did the crew work together? Were you all on the same page? If you were calling hand-checks, was everyone else calling hand-checks? Was there anywhere where you had to step between the official and the coach? Third, in the last two minutes was there a whistle that was warranted or was not warranted or that had an effect on the outcome of the game?"

These are three things that I'd want to know immediately. The officials I'm evaluating call me within 20 minutes of leaving the gym to go through this.

Feedback

We like to give feedback immediately. There are times when we don't want feedback from the coaches immediately, though. Often I'll say, "Let's talk tomorrow". Half the time they look at the video and see the official was right and there's no need to call me.

References

[1] Fédération Internationale de Football Association (FIFA). (2010). *Regulations on the Organisation of Refereeing in FIFA Member Associations*. Zürich, Switzerland: FIFA.
[2] MacMahon, C., Helsen, W. F., Starkes, J. L., & Weston, M. (2007). Decision-making skills and deliberate practice in elite association football referees. *Journal of Sports Sciences*, 25, 65–78.

[3] Biggs, A. (2006). Hackett plans to fast-track players into referees. *The Guardian*, online. http://www.guardian.co.uk/football/2006/jan/11/newsstory.sport4 (accessed 4 March 2011).

[4] James, S. (2006). Wanted: players to referee. *The Guardian*, online. http://www.guardian.co.uk/football/2006/feb/08/newsstory. sport7 (accessed 4 March 2011).

[5] Evans, G. (Ed.). (2004). *Problems and issues in the recruitment and retention of sports officials*. A report prepared for the Australian Sports Commission, Griffith University, Australia.

[6] Associate Press in The Hague. (2012). Dutch assistant referee dies after attack by teenage players. *The Guardian*, online. http://www.guardian.co.uk/football/2012/dec/04/dutch-assistant-referee-dies-attack-teenagers (accessed 17 April 2013).

[7] Titlebaum, P. J., Haberlin, N., & Titlebaum, G. (2009). Recruitment and retention of sports officials. *Recreational Sports Journal*, *33*, 102–8.

[8] Kellett, P., & Shilbury, D. (2007). Umpire participation: Is abuse really the issue? *Sport Management Review*, *10*, 209–29.

[9] Ericsson, K. A., Krampe, R. T., & Tesch-Romer, C. (1993). The role of deliberate practice in the acquisition of expert performance. *Psychological Review*, *100*, 363–406.

[10] Blake, C., Sherry, J., & Gissane, C. (2009). A survey of referee participation, training and injury in elite Gaelic game referees. *BMC Musculoskeletal Disorders*, *10*, 1–8.

[11] Krustrup, P., & Bangsbo, J. (2001). Physiological demands of top-class soccer refereeing in relation to physical capacity: effect of intense intermittent exercise training. *Journal of Sports Sciences*, *19*, 881–91.

[12] Weston, M., Helsen, W., MacMahon, C., & Kirkendall, D. (2004). The impact of specific high-intensity training sessions on football referees' fitness levels. *American Journal of Sports Medicine*, *32*(1, Suppl.), 54–61.

[13] Vickers, J. N. (Ed.). (2007). *Perception, cognition and decision training: The quiet eye in action*. Champaign, IL: Human Kinetics.

[14] Morris, P. H., & Lewis, D. (2010). Tackling diving: The perception of deceptive intentions in association football (soccer). *Journal of Nonverbal Behavior*, *34*, 1–13.

[15] Pizzera, A., & Raab, M. (2012). Does motor or visual experience enhance the detection of deceptive movements in football? *International Journal of Sports Science and Coaching*, *7*, 269–83.

[16] Renden, P. G., Kerstens, S., Oudejans, R. R. D., & Cañal-Bruland, R. (2012). Foul or dive? Motor contributions to judging ambiguous foul situations in football. *European Journal of Sport Science*, *14*(Suppl. 1), S221–7.

[17] Anshel, M. H., & Weinberg, R. S. (1999). Re-examining coping among basketball referees following stressful events: implications of coping interventions. *Journal of Sport Behavior*, *22*, 141–61.

[18] Catteeuw, P., Gilis, B., Jaspers, A., Wagemans, J., & Helsen, W. F. (2010). Training of perceptual-cognitive skills in offside decision making. *Journal of Sport and Exercise Psychology*, *32*, 845–61.

[19] Catteeuw, P., Gilis, B., Wagemans, J., & Helsen, W. F. (2010). Perceptual-cognitive skills in offside decision making: Expertise and training effects. *Journal of Sport and Exercise Psychology*, *32*, 828–44.

[20] Put, K., Wagemans, J., Jaspers, A., & Helsen, W. H. (2013). Web-based training improves on-field offside decision-making performance. *Psychology of Sport and Exercise*, *14*, 577–85.

[21] Brand, R., Plessner, H., & Schweizer, G. (2009). Conceptual considerations about the development of a decision-making training method for expert soccer referees. In D. Araújo, H. Ripoll, & M. Raab (Eds). *Perspectives on cognition and action in sport* (pp. 181–90). New York: Nova Science Publishers.

[22] Schweizer, G., Plessner, H., Kahlert, D., & Brand, R. (2011). A video-based training method for improving soccer referees' decision-making skills. *Journal of Applied Sport Psychology, 23*, 429–42.

[23] Mascarenhas, D. R. D., Collins, D., Mortimer, P. W., & Morris, B. (2005). Training accurate and coherent decision making in rugby union referees. *The Sport Psychologist, 19*, 131–47.

[24] MacMahon, C., Starkes, J. L., & Deakin, J. (2007). Referee decision making in a video-based infraction detection task: Application and training considerations. *International Journal of Sports Science & Coaching, 2*, 257 65.

[25] Anshel, M. H. (1995). Development of a rating scale for determining competence in basketball referees: Implications for sport psychology. *The Sport Psychologist, 9*, 4–28.

[26] Guillén, F., & Feltz, D. L. (2011). A conceptual model of referee efficacy. *Frontiers in Psychology, 2*, 1–5.

[27] Mascarenhas, D., Collins, D., & Mortimer, P. (2005). Elite refereeing performance: Developing a model for sport science support. *The Sport Psychologist, 19*, 364–79.

[28] Renton, P. (Ed.). (2012). *Panel Coaching Research Update*. Rugby Football Union technical report to the panel of referee coaches.

[29] Martin, J., Smith, N. C., Tolfrey, K., & Jones, A. M. (2001). Activity analysis of English premiership rugby football union refereeing. *Ergonomics, 44*, 1069–75.

10
CONCLUSION

Until now, science and knowledge about officiating has only been available in a very specific manner – that is, when officiating provides an interesting question in a discipline of study or when one sport focuses resources on the role. Thus, most often there is an isolated perspective, from only one sport, or examining only one aspect of the role, with little comparison with other sports. This book thus represents a major step forward by bringing together knowledge from different disciplines and different sports.

What we found in this approach, when examining the practice side of sports officiating, is a great sense of coherence. The Official's Call sections have been both enjoyable and informative. They provide reflection and highlight the important messages that resonate with officials. One of the striking things about these sections is that we often had to look back to confirm which specific chapter an official was commenting on, because they so frequently brought up content from one or several of the other chapters. This gives us the sense that the chapters are sound, which we were looking for. It also confirms that, whether they know it or not, the practitioners both use the science and are also clear examples of the science. As mentioned in the introduction in Chapter 1, this coherence is a characteristic of the early stages of a discipline of study.

There are also many signs in the previous chapters that, while officiating research is young, it is also a ripening discipline. For example, Chapter 2 provides a platform by presenting a more refined understanding of the different types of officials. This will help us to clarify precisely who, from the greater population of sports officials, any given piece of research addresses. Chapter 3 helps to reflect on how important physical demands can be in many sports. Not only this, it considers the connection between physical skills and decisions. Moreover, the Official's Call section by Bill

Mildenhall highlights that fitness can help a referee to deal with psychological pressure. Chapters 4 and 5 present complementary areas of visual perception and judgement and decision making. We saw that these are perhaps the areas with the most research base specific to officiating. Yet both chapters identified areas for continued work and many gaps in our knowledge. They also provide training considerations, which our officials picked up on and challenged. Chapter 6 addresses a particularly ripening area of work in discussing communication and game management, and draws on a diversity of disciplines, while Chapter 7 touches on the importance of psychological skills for officials, which, like Chapters 4 and 5, is also a more developed area. Chapter 8 addresses perhaps the fastest moving area and gives a more unified and structured perspective on the place of technology in officiating, which has been instrumental in training, which is considered in Chapter 9. The boundaries of this training and best approaches and expectations are a key area as we move forward, again signalling a ripening field.

The preceding chapters also make clear to us, however, that that there is a need to press forward and progress the science. While this book represents a huge step in this direction, more must be done to compare measures between sports and to increase the communication between referee associations from different sports. We must also progress towards understanding more complex problems, and exploring the hardest questions that we don't currently think we can answer. This progress will happen when the barriers to the research in this area, identified in Chapter 1, are addressed. One method of negotiating these barriers is to focus on producing interesting research. This is based on the fact that academics in sociology[1] and psychology[2] propose that, across disciplines, the research that produces the greatest lasting impact is, above all, *interesting*. We similarly propose that, for sports officiating, research that is interesting will attract more researchers and more funding, creating a groundswell for development and progress. Part of the definition of interesting research is that it may produce surprising results (e.g., the finding that elite athletes have no better basic vision or reaction times than their novice counterparts). From our point of view, this surprise and thus interest creates a greater likelihood of buy-in from both the science and practice sides of the sports officiating research equation. Supporting this, Davis[1] further defines interesting theories as those which not only challenge long-held beliefs and assumptions, but also have repercussions on both the theoretical and practical levels. This second part of the definition is particularly crucial for sports officiating research: the goal is to have an impact and ultimately improve practice.

The question is: how do we create more interesting practical work that has an impact? Kurt Gray and Daniel Wegner[2] propose six guidelines, two of which are particularly relevant for those in sports officiating research. The first is to focus on phenomena from everyday experiences. In Chapter 1 we discussed the difficulty of formulating 'good questions' from both the scientist's and practitioner's perspective. Gray and Wegner's first guideline helps to bridge this gap, and advises a focus on compelling experiences. An example from sports officiating is exploring a situation where athletes wearing red seem to be scored higher than similarly abled athletes in blue (as described in Chapter 5). This exploration captures a fascinating phenomenon: the power of performance-irrelevant features (colour) in borderline judgement situations. The identification of absorbing phenomena like this example requires a high level of immersion in the area to observe, remark and contemplate. Many researchers consider that they are immersed in sport as former or current athletes or spectators, or due to their overall love of sport. But true immersion, which reveals practice or occurrences beyond the assumed, or even a lack of familiarity which necessitates this immersion, may be the catalyst that is needed to spark key questions. An example of this method is the collaboration processes that were used in the early phases of a project in the similarly underdeveloped research area of dance. In one project,[3] scientists from multiple disciplines were immersed in a dance company to observe the processes used in choreographing and to formulate questions from their observations.[4,5] Researchers watched, recorded and noted while in the performance and rehearsal spaces. We thus encourage similar steps for immersion and discussion to identify phenomena with both theoretical and applied interest.

The second of Gray and Wegner's guidelines worthy of note for sports officiating research is the advice to formulate research designs that are engaging for participants. Designs which are more engaging to participate in are also more engaging to report, and thus to read, leading to greater excitement and interest, and hopefully the groundswell of more researchers and more funding. Luckily, officiating itself is a relatively engaging and complex area of research compared with many other topics such as basic skills in movement (reaching and grasping), perception (responses to relatively meaningless targets on a screen) or cognition (basic memory tests). Nevertheless, the more engaging we can make research designs, the better, especially when considering the remark by Gray and Wegner that ensuring that participants are engaged helps ensure more valid results.[2] Once again, open discussion between practitioners and scientists will help in this consideration of methodologies and design.

These steps to create interesting and engaging research may result in excellent smaller projects which contribute to the overall base and reach across sports. For example, from the contents of this book, we are prompted to ask:

- How generic are officiating skills in areas such as communication? Can they transfer between sports? How long would it take an expert basketball official to become an expert football official?
- Are there methods to improve our vision and decisions and attention that interact with technology? Is this desirable?
- Are there diminishing returns on training?
- How can we measure and train communication ability?
- Are there ways to standardise selection? Are there predictive models of who will make a good official, so we can select them earlier and they can thus participate longer?

It is also our task, given the state of the research, to identify the 'blue sky', ambitious and 'holy grail' questions. An example of an engaging but also central and challenging question in officiating was touched on both in Chapter 6 and in conversation with an elite official. At the NASO conference in 2009, a top basketball official with a distinguished career, who was then head of officiating, wanted to know: How good can I expect my officials to be? What are the limits? What total number of errors is acceptable; what's the top? A fascinating and seemingly intractable issue, it is undoubtedly a challenge, and quite possibly *the* challenge of the moment. However, it is also an example of one of the challenges that we envisage can be approached through aligning selection, training and education of referees between sports and countries more broadly. To understand how to optimise performance and professionalise the content as discussed in each chapter, we need actions such as centralising conferences, websites, stakeholder meetings in which the environment (rule books) and the key persons (referees) are discussed and the fit between task and competencies is optimised. Although there is a threat of descending into mere 'talk-fests', these sorts of actions have the potential to create the groundswell so clearly needed to progress the area, too long overlooked. Similar to the example of dance research that immersed researchers in the area, these centralising, focused actions in the area of officiating can be considered an immersion on a broader scale, to bring together officiating across sports and countries and progress the knowledge. Our hope is that this book can be, in some small way, a catalyst to these types of actions, as increased communication and collaboration will more clearly identify the most fruitful path forward.

References

[1] Davis, M.S. (1971). That's interesting!: Towards a phenomenology of sociology and a sociology of phenomenology. *Philosophy of the Social Sciences*, *1*, 309–44.

[2] Gray, K., & Wegner, D.M. (2013). Six guidelines for interesting research. *Perspectives on Psychological Science*, *8*, 549–53.

[3] deLahunta, S. (2009). The choreographic language agent. http://www.sdela.dds.nl/cla (accessed 21 May 2013).

[4] McGregor, W. Random dance. Aims and objectives. http://www.randomdance.org/r_research/aims_and_objectives (accessed 21 May 2013).

[5] McGregor, W. Random dance. Current projects. http://www.randomdance.org/r_research/current_projects1 (accessed 21 May 2013).

INDEX